Spirit
Baby

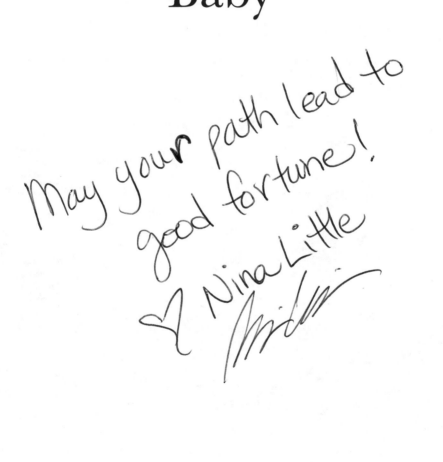

May your path lead to good fortune!

♡ Nina Little

Spirit Baby

TRAVELS THROUGH CHINA *on the*
LONG ROAD *to* MOTHERHOOD

Nina Neilson Little

ILLUMIFY MEDIA GLOBAL
Littleton, Colorado

Spirit
Baby

Published by
Illumify Media Global
www.IllumifyMedia.com
"Write. Publish. Market. *SELL!*"

Library of Congress Control Number: 2019932347

Paperback ISBN: 978-1-949021-45-5
eBook ISBN: 978-1-949021-46-2

Printed in the United States of America

To my Spirit Baby, who gave me hope, and to the country of China, which gave me strength. You will forever remain in my heart.

CONTENTS

ACKNOWLEDGMENTS

I would like to express my appreciation and love for my husband, Chris, who walked beside me on my journey to motherhood and to becoming an author; my mother, who has stood by me throughout my life; and my sisters and children, who have greatly enriched my life.

In addition, I would like to express my gratitude for my acupuncturist and friend, Deborah Skelton of Twin Cranes Natural Healing Center, who helped me to heal in many ways. I would like to thank Dr. Mark Bush at Conceptions Reproductive Associates for helping me to survive infertility.

I would also like to thank my writing partner, Melanie Kallai, and friends, Ashley Seifert and Emily Koechel, who supported me throughout this memoir writing process. And lastly, I would like to thank my editor, Karen Scalf Bouchard, who was truly my "book midwife."

Thank you all for believing in me, supporting me, and helping to make this dream possible.

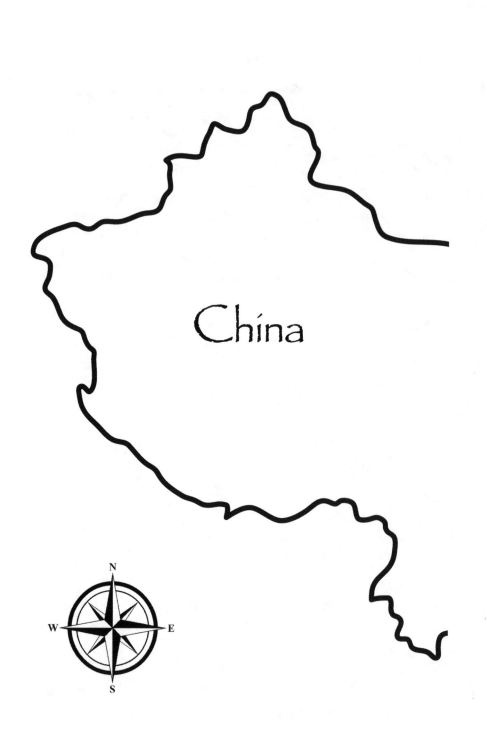

China

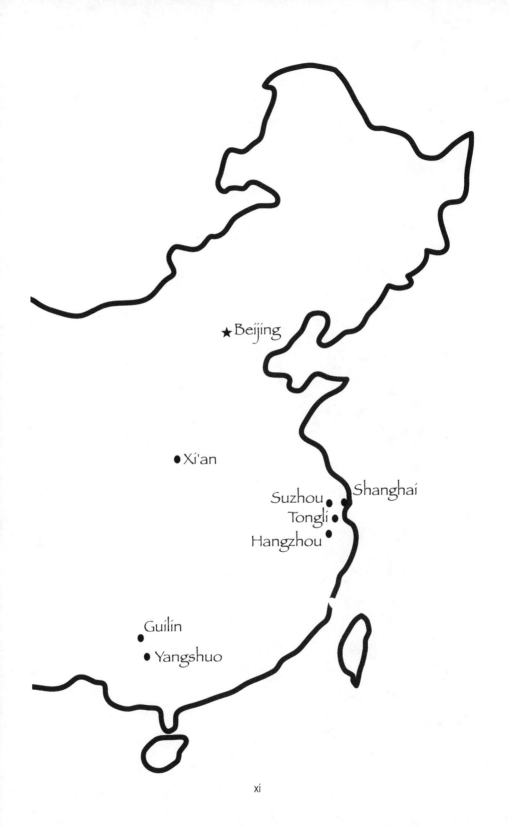

★Beijing

●Xi'an

Suzhou● ●Shanghai
Tongli●
Hangzhou●

Guilin
●
●Yangshuo

INTRODUCTION

"Hey Lady, you want dog? You like!" is not a question I ever expected to hear.

As my husband and I navigated through the chaos on Wangfujing Snack Street past colorful stalls displaying a variety of exotic snacks, mostly on sticks, the air was filled with pungent smells and curious sounds. In addition to the noisy banter of the vendors touting their specialties and inviting passersby to try tantalizing samples of insects, reptiles, and sea creatures, we heard a dizzying mélange of foreign languages.

We had arrived in Beijing just in time for the notorious spring sand storms. Every year massive clouds of yellow Mongolian sand wreak havoc throughout East Asia, reducing visibility and air quality in China's capital city to hazardous levels.

And, like the swirling Gobi Desert, I had a volatile, emotional storm brewing within me.

At thirty-five, I assumed I would be happily raising a family in the suburbs, not traveling through China and being coaxed to eat dog by vendors at a nighttime street market. (Not that I would ever consider eating dog. After struggling for years to have children, my dog, Otis, was my surrogate baby. However, on a street corner in Beijing, my husband and I did share our first snake on a stick—it tasted like a saltier, greasier version of chicken.)

I would love to claim our trip to China as one of the backpacking, youth hostel, shoestring-budget adventures of my youth, but that would be a lie. This was the luxury getaway of a married couple in their mid-thirties trying to escape from the anguish of failed fertility treatments, the heartbreak of another miscarriage, and the silence of our empty, childless home.

We'd started trying to have a family four years earlier. During that time, my husband and I had made traveling after pregnancy failures our top coping mechanism, selling stocks, cashing in bonds, and maxing out credit cards in pursuit of the cathartic release we felt while traveling. Traveling had given us a reprieve from our suffering by allowing us to alter our reality and find some joy in our existence. It was also a way for us to make the most of our "dual income, no kids" status. While literally all our friends and family were busy making babies, we stayed sane by traveling to exotic locations. While our friends sent out birth announcements and holiday cards featuring blissful families, we sent out cards with photos of us on top of volcanoes, hanging from zip lines, and lounging on the beach (me in a bikini with no stretch marks).

Of course, nothing had truly dulled the pain we felt over not being able to have a family.

According to my acupuncturist and Chinese herbalist, there's an ancient Chinese belief that women possess two hearts: an upper heart associated with the standard Western organ as well as a lower heart tied to the uterus. Based on this philosophy, women hold dreams of infants, lost children, and babies that were never meant to be in their upper hearts, while babies destined to be born travel to their mother's lower heart.

My upper heart was full of lost babies and broken dreams. But the promise of a Chinese baby girl was beginning to fill my upper heart with hope.

After two very long, painful years of infertility struggles and treatments, my husband, Chris, and I decided on an adoption program through China. We signed endless official contracts; submitted essays attesting to our sound mental states, financial stability, and desire to become parents; were reviewed multiple times by Social Services; invested several thousand dollars; and began the long, hard wait toward adoption of a baby girl from China.

Starting the adoption process awakened me from a deeply depressed, trance-like, hopeless state by giving me a sense of direction and promise. I was convinced that adopting a baby would put an end to my suffering. While I still felt the pain of not being able to conceive a child and held onto the hope that one day I might have a biological child as well, I was excited to embrace another culture and thereby enrich my world. In lieu of creating a life, I hoped I would forge a unique bond through adoption with a child, both of us lost, in pain, and in need of each other.

Suddenly my life had a new purpose—to learn everything I could about the history, language, and customs of China so that I could become a culturally aware and sensitive parent to an adopted Chinese orphan. I turned into a crazy, white lady obsessed with China. I read the works of Chinese authors, both old and new. I shopped in Asian markets, ate at dim sum buffets, and visited Asian bath houses. I volunteered as an English tutor for Asian immigrants. I attended local festivals celebrating the Chinese New Year, as well as, Lantern and Dragon Boat Festivals. I decorated my generic, middle-class home in a mostly white neighborhood in suburban Denver with Chinese lanterns and banners to drive away bad luck during Chinese holidays.

For a while, I managed to hide from the pain, stress, and fear of infertility by encapsulating myself inside a Chinese bubble. I put up a brave front against the perils of infertility, but the Herculean effort took its toll. We continued to try to conceive while waiting to adopt, and as the weeks turned to months, I started to waver and lose hope in both medical technology and international adoption.

We decided to take a break. I needed to escape from the stacks of books on adopting a high-needs orphan. I longed for a reprieve from hormone drugs and sleepless nights researching infertility treatments on the Internet. I was sick from the endless hours of weeping, watching reruns of *Friends*, and eating nachos. I needed to get away from the pile of negative pregnancy tests filling up the wastebasket and the phone, which still hadn't rung with the message to "come get your baby."

I had reached the brink of despair. That's when we bought plane tickets and fled to China . . . and she saved my life.

1

TOUCH THE STONES

Life moved very fast in Beijing, and it was easy to get overwhelmed. My first impression was that Chinese people appeared to dwell in a state of perpetual motion. But while they seemed to have a harmonious rhythm, we stood out and disrupted the flow. We were strangers in a crowded, fast-paced, extraordinary land filled with promise and wonder.

On our first night in China, Chris and I ventured out alone on the congested sidewalks of Beijing. I was immediately struck by the number of bicycles. They clogged the sidewalks, blocked doorways, and overflowed into the streets, competing with cars and pedestrians.

We saw bicycle-powered fresh fruit stands and flower shops. We observed a man riding a bicycle with a mobile barber shop in tow, complete with large mirrors; a red velvet chair; and an antique red, white, and blue-striped barber pole. A passerby flagged him down and got a spur-of-the-moment haircut on the side of the road, from a presumable stranger, in the near dark.

Everywhere we looked, there were small shops, street vendors, and even more bicycles pulling carts offering every snack you could possibly imagine, round the clock.

For a street market, Wangfujing Snack Street was extremely organized and efficient with rows of metal stands neatly lined on one side of the wide avenue. The stands were equipped with red-and-white striped fabric roofs, red curtains along the open backsides, and menu panels along the tops of the roofs. Vendors in matching long, white-collared shirts with red aprons and visors, and very official-looking photo ID badges, looked more like barbers from the 1950s than food vendors.

As we explored the snack street, I'd like to say I was curious, excited, and feeling brave, but in truth I was overwhelmed and apprehensive. As we wandered past stalls offering squid, whole baby sharks, starfish, centipedes, seahorses, scorpions, silkworms, and giant beetles on bamboo skewers (and the aforementioned dog), our conversation reflected the culture shock we were experiencing:

"What do you suppose *that* is?"

"How the hell do you eat a sea urchin—start with the butt?"

"Gross, don't look at its eyes!"

"I dare you to eat that huge, hairy tarantula!"

To my great relief, there were also stalls with more familiar fare such as dumplings, noodles, beef balls, crabs, various flavors of fried rice, and egg rolls. Just about everything was served with Chinese Five Spice Powder, a blend of cloves, peppercorns, fennel, cinnamon, and star anise, which offered the sour, bitter, pungent, sweet-and-spicy flavors of China in perfect balance.

The local culinary options, as unfamiliar as they were, presented a welcomed reprieve from my faithful following of a fertility-boosting diet, and my manic focus on protein consumption. For four years, I'd eaten insane quantities of nuts and a wide variety of beans (single-handedly dispelling the rumor that beans cause flatulence—or maybe I simply built up a tolerance). I had happily consumed avocados with gusto, had no qualms avoiding mercury-filled sea creatures, and obediently downed sea kelp. I'd eaten thousands of eggs for a literal and symbolic fertility boost. I'd stopped drinking coffee and consumed tea instead; this and no margaritas were the ultimate sacrifice.

While in China I completely rejected my fertility diet and ate with reckless abandon, cultural curiosity, and pure enjoyment. That first night Chris and I sampled beef, shrimp, and snake on a stick. Since there were no tables, we ate our dinner on the curb.

For dessert, there were sticks stacked with colorful assortments of candied fruit, the most traditional being Chinese hawthorn. Known as *tanghulu*, the kabob-style sticks of giant strawberries, triangles of pineapple, and green and orange squares of melon looked exquisite. But thanks to the rock-hard candy syrup coating, they seemed unappetizing and a bit too much like the fake fruit adorning dinner tables in a Pottery Barn catalog. However, I enjoyed watching a toddler in a stroller attempt to eat a strawberry as big as his fist (and holler when it fell to the ground and was snatched up by a bird).

We were highly entertained by three Australian guys in their mid-twenties who were daring each other to eat a scorpion to impress their cheering girlfriends. One managed to bite off the tail of a large, shiny, black scorpion. Then, he promptly spewed it onto the ground, smashed it with his foot and yelled, "I am the Scorpion King!" This garnered applause from the girlfriends and a combination of high fives, slaps on the back, and chest bumps from his mates. It wasn't long before the two remaining adventurous gourmands caved to peer pressure (and their male egos) and followed suit.

The spectacle caused several food vendors to roll their eyes, jab each other in the ribs, and shake their heads, while Chris simply muttered "morons" under his breath. I wondered if the Australians had been offered any dog.

$$\text{❀}$$

A woman who longs for a child doesn't need a reason. She doesn't need to have suffered through a disjointed childhood or have grown up feeling displaced to long desperately to marry, conceive, and finally create a close-knit, stable family of her own.

But you must admit, that's a damn good reason.

I should know.

The first ten years of my life I was a sad, lonely, only child. My parents divorced when I was a toddler, and I was shuffled back and forth between two completely opposite homes. I became two different daughters. I acted one way around my open-minded, free-spirited mother in laid-back Santa Fe, New Mexico and another around my intimidating, career-driven father in cosmopolitan Denver, Colorado. I was what you might call a poor little rich girl.

During the school year, I lived with my bi-polar, artist and elementary school teacher mother, who wore thrift-store fashions and drove a beat-up station wagon covered in liberal bumper stickers. We lived in an artist commune; shopped at an organic co-op; and frequented yoga ashrams, art festivals, and spiritual seminars.

I also wore brand-name clothes, attended elite private school summer camps, and took vacations to Europe and the Caribbean—thanks to my wealthy father. But my father wasn't a regular presence in my life. I only saw him during holidays and summers, and even then I spent most of my time with the hired help. Immediately upon my arrival, my summer governess, my father's secretary, or his latest girlfriend would take me to be "de-hippie-fied." They would have my hair cut into a pristine bob, my nails manicured, and completely overhaul my wardrobe. I was primped, preened, and ready for display during the few times my father found having a well-mannered, smart and subservient daughter to be beneficial to his business endeavors (and the rest of the time I was invisible).

My father was a virtual stranger and was mostly neglectful, often critical, and always distant. As a real estate developer, he took huge risks for potential financial gain and was always working the next deal. The only times I saw him relax were while piloting his airplane or after a few Jack Daniels. The only things we had in common were a love of skiing and dogs. My relationship with my father was so strained and uncomfortable that as a child I used to listen in the mornings for the sound of the garage door opening underneath my bedroom, watch my father's red Jaguar back down the driveway, and only then head downstairs for breakfast. The few times we had breakfast together, my father would simply read the *Wall Street Journal,* or we would awkwardly talk about the weather.

The one time my high-brow father deigned to visit New Mexico, which he described as "only slightly less depressing, hot, and dirty than a Mexican prison," I couldn't wait to prove to my doubting classmates that my father was sophisticated, affluent, and most of all legit. He came to my third-grade class to give a slideshow on Kenya, where one of his fraternity brothers owned a stately coffee plantation and we had spent a summer after my parents' divorce. I was completely mortified that instead of his standard Brooks Brothers suit and tie, he showed up wearing a tribal robe and carrying a spear. While my father showed pictures of me sitting in a helicopter and petting an orphaned pet zebra, I wished I could have crawled under a rock. After the presentation I insisted he remove his robe and then proceeded to parade him around the cafeteria at lunchtime, so everyone could see my father in his custom-tailored suit, complete with a monogramed handkerchief and silk tie.

I was desperate to fit in and find my place in life. Growing up, I was an anomaly: the shy, nerdy tomboy with a bohemian mom and a millionaire dad, and my classmates didn't know what to make of me or what to believe. I hardly knew what to think of myself.

Like all of us, my childhood experiences, my personal stories have shaped me. Nations have stories, too. Perhaps my struggle with my own narrative was the very thing that made me so enamored with the history I felt all around me, the enthralling history which helped to shape the incredible country of China. Then again, who wouldn't be fascinated by Zhongguo, the Middle Kingdom, the center of civilization (at least according to the ancient Chinese).

When we arrived in Beijing, our first tour guide was a young woman named Zhao Rui. Her name meant "one who encourages others," and it couldn't have been more appropriate. For her foreign clients, however, she chose to go by the name Laura. She was tiny, adorable, and delightfully talkative, with hands half the size of my own. We set off together on a grand tour of the many historical sites of Beijing, starting with a visit to China's most famous landmark: The Great Wall.

In a word, the Great Wall of China was "breathtaking," since both "heart-stopping" and "awe-inspiring" are technically two words. But in truth, there are no words to describe my reaction to seeing the Great Wall—something I had seen many times in books, on TV, and featured in calendars at the dentist's office—up close and in person.

The sheer magnitude of the wall was staggering. Even after twenty-seven hundred years of deterioration, the fortress wall stretched fifty-five hundred miles. The network of walls, which were built in stages over roughly twenty dynasties, once spanned 13,170 miles, nearly half the size of the circumference of the Earth's equator. But statistics fail to adequately describe the incredible feat of engineering, and I, a writer, am left with no words.

"It's like this," Laura told us. "The northside of the wall is higher and stronger because the enemy came from the north, while the southside is lower and has access doors." She added, "In former times, the watchtowers were filled with grain, supplies, and sleeping quarters. And the smokestacks on top of each tower were used to warn of invaders. One smoke signal meant five hundred soldiers, and two smoke signals meant one thousand invaders. Villagers would steal the granite bricks, which were high quality and sealed with only glutinous rice flour, for their homes."

The Great Wall served as a protective shield, guarding the capital and imperial temples for generations from northern nomads, but ultimately it failed to protect t' e Han people from established northern tribes. In 1279, Kublai Khan crushed the Song dynasty resistance and established the Yuan dynasty, and in 1644 the Manchus invaded and brought down the Ming dynasty. So in the end, the Great Wall was one of history's greatest exercises in futility.

As I walked atop the ancient fortress, I was most impressed by the view of a vast, jagged, mountain range and the staggering height, width, and length of the mighty wall. But instead of focusing on the arduous efforts of the Chinese to protect themselves from invasion, I found myself pondering the determination of the legions who attempted to scale the wall. I thought about the many obstacles I'd already overcome on this long road to motherhood and how, if necessary, I would scale the Great Wall of China— like a crazed Mongol overlord—to get a baby.

After more than a year of the natural method with no pregnancy, my husband and I had been poked, prodded, tested, and analyzed. One of my fallopian tubes was "Roto-Rootered" to clear out some random tissue build up and the sperm analysis came back slightly wonky, but none of the findings were considered serious. Roughly 40 percent of infertility was believed to be male factor, while another 40 percent was thought to be female factor and the remaining was unexplained—we fell into the unexplained category.

We went through three rounds of intrauterine insemination, or IUI (aka, the turkey baster method), with the intense egg production stimulation drug Clomid . . . with no results. We did a round of in-vitro fertilization, or IVF, with the implantation of one embryo . . . with no results. We followed this with a second round of IVF and the implantation of two frozen embryos. One took and I became pregnant but soon miscarried.

About one out of every three IVF cycles is successful. Therefore, after each attempt the two weeks we had to wait until I could take a pregnancy test were the longest and most stressful of my entire life.

Upon learning my first IVF attempt failed, I cried like I had never cried before. I cried as if all previous crying had been the pouty, fake blubbering of a spoiled toddler, and this was the real deal, an expression of true pain and unfathomable anguish. I took ugly crying to a new level with convulsive, hyperventilating, delirious sobbing. My floodgates burst wide open, and my body simply let go. I cried until there were no tears left, and I was dry as a desert and then I wept some more. I entered a state of complete shock and disbelief, as I desperately tried to understand how a young, healthy woman with good eggs couldn't conceive a child.

After getting pregnant from my second round of IVF, then losing the baby, I became hysterical, completely unhinged and volatile. I moaned and screamed like I was possessed by the devil himself. I cursed my creator, my flawed body, and the concept of fate. I took my copy of *What to Expect When You're Expecting*, my unfinished pregnancy journal, and a pile of baby supplies and dumped them on the floor of the nursery closest—and slammed the door. I couldn't believe after all my suffering, I had been given a glimpse of motherhood, only to experience it slowly perish within me.

By the time I went for a D&C to remove the nonviable fetus, I had gone to a very dark place. I was beyond depressed and over and above despondent. I became completely numb and was simply going through the motions like a brain-dead zombie. I had given up. I was hopeless, faithless, and utterly lost.

These painful memories disrupted my reverie as I stood atop the Great Wall. The long road that had led us to China had been filled with dashed hopes, loss, and grief. Gazing across the hills, an undulating sea of yellows, greens, and browns in early spring, I tried to push away the melancholy that had followed me even here, halfway around the world.

Laura was saying something. Lost in thought, I snapped back to the present, in time to hear some wise advice.

"You must reach out and touch the stones," she said encouragingly. "We have a saying that 'You are not a hero until you climb the Great Wall.' Don't just look with your eyes, you must touch the stones and feel the history."

Most people who know me would agree that, under normal circumstances, I'm bold and adventurous. But lately I'd been plagued by anxiety and despair. I felt like anything but a hero.

I wondered if climbing the Great Wall and touching the stones of history would mark the beginning of something new. Was I ready to stop wallowing in depression and rejoin the living? The idea of making some new memories, feeling ancient history, and perhaps rewriting some of my own story resonated within my soul, something that had been dormant for too long. It was time to touch some stones.

On the two-hour car ride back to Beijing, Laura and I talked nonstop. For one thing, she had recently gotten engaged and asked us for all sorts of marital advice.

What I wanted to say was, "Don't be infertile, since guilt, anxiety, and a methodical love life would surely take their toll on any marriage, especially a new one. It takes a seriously strong marital bond to survive the throes of infertility, so my wish for any, new couple who wants children is for a free pass to abundance."

Of course, I wasn't about to share these kinds of heavy sentiments with my freshly engaged new friend. Instead, I smiled and told Laura I was more interested in hearing about Chinese wedding traditions, both ancient and modern, and she was happy to oblige.

According to Laura, a month or so before a wedding, the bride celebrates her "cookie day," when the groom's family sends food and gifts to "sweeten" the loss of a daughter. The cookies are delivered in large, red Double Happiness boxes, together with other snacks representing the Wu Fu, or five blessings of prosperity, happiness, longevity, many children, and peace.

Laura said a Chinese bride traditionally wore no shoes and was carried by the groom, while her mother carried her shoes. This custom symbolized the responsibility of raising a daughter and holding her in your hands. Changing shoes was an old belief that the bride should not bring earth on the soles of her shoes from her parent's home into her new home, since her previous life should be left behind.

(I'm embarrassed to admit that shortly after learning of this tradition, I purchased a tiny pair of red, silk, baby slippers and placed them under my pillow—being truly desperate, slightly insane, and willing to try anything—to show my commitment to motherhood.)

Laura told us that traditionally the bride was covered with a scarf with the image of a dragon on it to dispel evil spirits and was likely sobbing hysterically to demonstrate her love for her parental home. For good measure, a brazier of charcoal and fire was set at the entrance to the groom's family's home, and the bride had to jump over the brazier so that evil spirits would not follow her.

"It's like this," she said. "Women have yin, associated with night and dark, so spirits follow women. It could be a good spirit that protects her, but when she goes to the husband's home, he takes care of her and the ghost must leave."

In addition, the bride was expected to serve her in-laws tea to symbolize becoming part of the family. The new couple searched the wedding suite for "hidden ghosts," wedding guests playing an embarrassing prank and children who were encouraged to frolic on the bed to bless the impending nuptials. If that wasn't enough subtle innuendo, the newlyweds slept upon a bed of nuts, dates, and longan fruit, which symbolized the prompt birth of a son.

I wondered if my infertility issues were due to the fact that I hadn't jumped over a fire filled brazier to the entrance of my husband's home upon marriage and had royally pissed off my yin ghost. Plus, I've never made my in-laws tea, invited toddlers to jump on my bed, nor tried sleeping on a layer of trail mix.

Throughout my life, countless people have asked me how my polar opposite parents became a couple. My token response is that they were cut from the same cloth—upper-class Texas society. My mother's family was in the law and my father's family was in the oil business. When my parents met, my father had recently received his law degree, and my mother was nice looking, well bred, and just so happened to be the daughter of a supreme court justice for the State of Texas. It should have been a perfect match—at least in theory, and according to the Junior League and the society pages.

Frankly, I'm glad my parents divorced. My father was born with a silver spoon in his mouth and remained a true elitist who was obsessed with his career and finances. Meanwhile, my mother left high society behind, moved to the Land of Enchantment, and found her true self as an artist. Santa Fe was a wonderful place to grow up. I was wild and free and far from the confines of my upper-class lineage, at least nine months out of the year.

My life changed dramatically when both my parents remarried, and I became the big sister to three half sisters. My two half sisters from my mother's marriage are ten and eleven years younger than me and, due to my stepfather's Italian heritage, significantly darker skinned and shorter than I am. As a result, people regularly assumed I was their Swedish or German nanny. My half sister from my father's marriage is fifteen years younger and looks just like me. People often mistook me for her mother.

I adore my half sisters and am happier not being an only child, but due to my significantly different age and appearance, and my siblings' favored status I often felt a bit like the misfit Cinderella (minus the never-ending chores and talking animals). As stepparents go, mine weren't too bad, certainly not within legendary evil stepparent range, but still I learned to keep my place and hide amongst the shadows.

The dynamic within my mother's home consisted of two teams: my stepfather and two stepsisters versus me and my mom. Through no fault of my sisters—they were just children—the world revolved around them, and I was left to fend for myself. My stepfather lavished attention on his children, gave little affection to my mother, and completely ignored me. I felt invisible and without my mother's love would have completely disappeared. My mother and I were a team. We weren't perfect, but we always had each other's backs when the shit got real.

Meanwhile, my father continued to neglect me. I was, however, my stepmother's little pet. She used to take me shopping for clothes, to movies, and to nail salons, until she had a daughter of her own. Still, we continued to get along just fine, until the lawsuit.

Early on, my father had stopped paying child support, and for years my mother had made do without his money—until it was time for me to go to college. That's when my mom offered my father a great deal: the opportunity to pay for his honor-roll daughter to go to an in-state university in lieu of coughing up a hefty amount of back child support. He refused. Ultimately, my mom sued. My college tuition was paid for, but my relationship with half my family was ruined.

My stepmother claimed I was a traitor and began referring to my mother by a wide variety of colorful words. My relationship with my stepmother might have survived if she hadn't destroyed my basic accord with my father, kept me from my little sister, and caused me to be fully disinherited. (Come to think of it, maybe she qualifies for legendary evil stepmother status, after all!)

Ultimately, my father had three children with three different wives, divorced his first two wives, and disowned his first two children, including myself and my older half brother. Since both my brother and I chose to live with our mothers, we grew up apart, in different states, with different families. I met my brother three times when I was just a child. I know little more of him than his name. He's one of many lost pieces of my broken family.

My original birth family fell apart, and I didn't fit within my two, new stepfamilies. I grew up thinking I didn't belong anywhere. The feeling of being a misfit, an extra, and an outsider haunted me. I was desperate to find my place in the world.

I hoped that as a wife and mother I would feel like I was an integral part of something; that I would finally be forever included, needed, and loved; that I would finally have a genuine home. As a mother—the queen bee—I hoped to finally have a starring, not a supporting, role in my own life.

There's something about traveling to an unfamiliar place—full of challenges and new discoveries—that can provide you with whatever you are searching for. Do you need a new perspective on your life? Traveling will gift it to you. Do you need healing?

You can find that too. Nightlife and adventure? Solitude and relaxation? You can discover it all in the world beyond your front door.

While traveling did not make a baby appear out of thin air, it reawakened my curiosity and desire to learn. Plus, it gave me an unexpected gift: a newfound appreciation for my unusual name, something I had disliked for decades until I learned, in China, how powerful it is.

While touring the stunning Temple of Heaven, built in 1420, I observed a reoccurring architectural theme.

The Circular Mound Altar is a three-layered altar made of marble. It is where the winter solstice ceremonies were held. Each of the layers is divided by nine steps. The lowest layer was created for the people, the middle layer was designated for the ancestors, and the top layer was reserved for the gods. The altar is enclosed by two walls: the inner one is circular and higher, symbolizing heaven, and the outer one is square and lower, symbolizing the earth. At winter solstice, the emperor stood in the center to pray upon the Heaven Heart Stone, surrounded by a brick pattern in multiples of nine that helped raise his voice to heaven as he prayed for good weather, bountiful harvests, and luck for the people.

I asked Laura about the significance of the number nine and multiples of nine in Chinese architectural design, explaining that I had a personal interest due to my name.

Throughout the world, my name is pronounced Nēna. However, I was given the less common pronunciation of Nīna. I have never much cared for my name and the fact that it rhymes with the number nine, nor that I was named after an ancestor who after her husband died from the plague married her husband's brother. As early as kindergarten, kids began to call me Nina Vagina. By high school my nickname became Nina-210, (after a popular TV show at the time, *Beverly Hills 90210*) and in college it progressed to Sixty-Nina (use your imagination).

I was elated when I saw that, in China, the number nine is revered.

Laura explained that the number nine has the same pronunciation as the Chinese word *jiŭ*, meaning everlasting. Nine is also the luckiest number because it is complete, as the highest single-digit number in base 10 and contains characteristics of all the lower numbers. To the ancient Chinese, nine was the largest number pertaining to man, as numbers ten and above belonged to heaven. Therefore, nine was reserved solely for the emperor. Chinese emperors wore nine dragon imperial robes and ordered the construction of nine dragon walls and other design elements in relationship with and in multiples of the number nine to show their great power, hope for longevity, and eternal reign of their empire.

Still thinking of her words, I climbed the steps of the Hall of Prayer for Good Harvests. As I did, my eyes filled with tears, my heart raced, and I felt a sense of serenity. I truly felt as though I were experiencing an emotional awakening. The focal point of the Temple of Heaven complex was a masterpiece of wood frame construction, built with no nails or beams, only interconnected rafters and sets of symbolic columns. The round temple, on a white marble platform, had three layers of eaves each covered with blue-colored glaze symbolizing heaven. The layered eaves created the sensation of rising up to the promised land.

The central hall featured a flat, circular, marble design called the dragon and phoenix stone. According to legend, originally the stone had only a phoenix, while there was a dragon pattern on the ceiling. As time went by, the dragon and the phoenix fell in love and eventually became one. The pairing of dragons and phoenix can be seen throughout China, as the two creatures represent the emperor and empress and a balanced, perfect union.

Laura insisted that Chris and I stop for a kiss upon the stone for good luck and the token cheesy photo op. When we kissed, I could almost remember what life for us had been like before the longing for illusive babies had completely taken over.

Later, while exploring the once Forbidden City, I was delighted to discover more architectural elements in multiples of nine.

Now known as the Palace Museum and open to the public since 1949, the complex was the exclusive domain of twenty-four emperors and the political center of China for almost five hundred years. Constructed from 1406 to 1420, at the central axis of old Beijing, the palace consists of 980 buildings and covers 178 acres. It was long believed to have 9,999 rooms, the ultimate in number nine luckiness, but actually has a mere 8,704 rooms. The three main halls all have a height of nine *zhang* and nine *chi* (ancient Chinese units of measurement), as well as eighty-one doornails in nine rows and nine columns on each gate. The number of almost all the stairs is nine or a multiple of nine.

While strolling around the Forbidden City, Laura told us a rather scandalous story about the emperor's late-night habits. The Hall of Heavenly Purity had nine identical bedrooms, so no one could tell the emperor from his fakes.

"Many nights, the eunuchs would check naked concubines for weapons, then roll them up in a carpet and take them to the emperor's quarters," she said. "Then they would push the carpet and shut the door before it completed unrolling."

According to Laura, the eunuchs lived in three-sided courtyards, always without a fourth side, to represent what they were missing (geez, way to rub salt in the wound).

It was exhilarating, seeing things in a new light and finding beauty and significance in what had been ignored, misunderstood, or considered mundane. My name means everlasting and symbolizes completeness—and that's not something to be taken lightly.

My inability to carry a child had left me weak and insecure.

Could China help me find my strength and confidence once more?

2

FOO DOGS
AND TIGER MOMS

When we first arrived in Beijing, we noticed a yellowish-brown smog, which suggested a recent disaster such as a volcanic eruption, a massive fire, or the fallout from a nuclear bomb. But it was merely the annual, spring dust storms created by the Gobi Desert just north of the capital. While many fear the Mongolian desert will one day swallow Beijing in its entirety, we were treated to surprisingly pleasant weather, with only a slight haze. Due to several windy days immediately before our arrival in mid-March, we were given an unexpected reprieve from the high rates of pollution and seasonal sand storms. (To my great relief, I did not have to wear an ugly respirator mask and was not completely dependent on my asthma inhaler.)

We celebrated the lovely spring weather with a casual stroll around the enchanting Beihai Park, which borders the northern edge of the Forbidden City. The park featured an enormous lake, several islands, numerous pavilions, rock gardens, bamboo forests, a Buddhist temple and a 120-foot white stupa. The park was opened to the public in 1925 after being an imperial garden for more than one thousand years.

The air was filled with the intoxicating scent of jasmine. As Chris and I walked, we saw chrysanthemums and peonies the size of my head. Showers of white and soft pink plum blossoms fell from the heavens. It was unbelievably charming and romantic. We held hands and kissed, like we used to—before trying to have a baby had turned us into romantically challenged robots.

Kissing my husband had long been one of my favorite activities, despite the fact that our first kiss was delayed by a comedy of errors. On my third date with Chris, at a Mexican restaurant in Boulder well known for its potent margaritas, I got completely drunk (on a single margarita). This was particularly embarrassing since margaritas are my favorite drink, and I've often claimed to have a high tolerance for tequila. Chris was a complete gentleman and drove me to my apartment in my beat-up Subaru. If he had intended on snuggling, my dog, Jane—a yellow lab mix that I'd rescued from the pound—did not give him the option. She followed his every move, growling protectively as he tucked me in. Later, when he came to check on me and sat down on the bed, Jane barfed on him. She lay down across the bed next to me while Chris slept on the couch by default. Our first kiss had to wait until the following morning while we were taking Jane for a walk in the foothills, through fields of wild flowers. It was worth the wait.

The entrance to the Chanfu Buddhist temple housed the Four Heavenly Kings, a set of guardian statues representing the four directions, which we soon learned were prominently featured within every Buddhist temple in China. Laura informed us that the chief and protector of the north, heard everything, controlled wealth and held an umbrella that opened and then trapped evil spirits inside. The king of the south, who ruled over the wind, caused roots to grow and held a sword that symbolized power over ignorance. The king of the west, who saw all, held a venomous snake with the curing medicine in his opposite hand. Lastly, the king of the east and God of music upheld the realm and made beautiful melodies with a pipa instrument to convert listeners to Buddhism.

While visiting the Chengguang Hall, Laura said, "It's like this, the Buddhas of the Han people are colorful and realistic, while Tibetan Buddhas are golden. The Buddha to the West represents past life, the Buddha in the center is for present life, and the Buddha in the East symbolizes the next life."

I thought about my hopes and dreams for my present and future life. I told Laura about our struggles with infertility and our hopes to adopt a Chinese orphan one day. I felt relieved when the Chinese national responded with enthusiasm and support for our foreign adoption. She said, "I know your karma is good by how you treat others kindly and care about children. I know you have much interest in learning about China since you ask lots of questions and write in your notebook. So you will be a good mother to a Chinese baby." I hugged her and cried a little on her shoulder.

We walked along ornate, curved bridges through the Five-Dragon Pavilions, consisting of five connected pavilions with spires and upswept eaves. From a distance, the structures appeared to blend together and resembled a giant, twisting dragon skimming the water.

A large group of adorable Chinese schoolchildren on a field trip paraded past in neat, straight lines, wearing matching red uniforms and coats. Laura informed us that all Chinese students wore uniforms to school. First, for safety, as a quick and easy way to identify where each child attended school. Second, for uniformity to cut down on teasing and jealousy. She added, "The uniforms were thin and cheap, and I remember being very cold as a student in the winter."

As I looked at their smiling, happy faces, I searched for the image of my future Chinese daughter amongst them, even if only a vague concept from my dreams. The sight of chubby-cheeked children was about to bring on the waterworks, when a young Chinese mother suddenly approached me and literally handed me her baby girl. Laura quickly explained that it was widely believed that a baby would have good luck if held by a white Westerner. To my surprise, the baby did not cry, and the mother, Chris, and several bystanders took our picture. Rather than feeling jealous at this mother's joy, I felt truly honored and a new sense of happiness and peace came over me. If only I had known how to do a proper Western blessing.

As a mostly vegetarian, newly and only slightly carnivorous, and very picky eater, I was apprehensive about dining in China. Would the meat be undercooked? Would every meal be insanely spicy or ridiculously sweet? Would the food be intolerably bizarre and include cat and dog meat or monkey brains? Would I become deathly ill from some Chinese form of extreme tummy distress, a.k.a. Chairman Mao's Revenge? It turned out for the most part the food throughout China was absolutely delicious. After a few days of eating cautiously, avoiding meat and anything fried, I threw caution to the wind and thoroughly enjoyed (almost) every meal. Fertility diet be dammed!

Every morning, our hotel in Beijing served a Western-style Chinese buffet in a giant ballroom with the soundtrack to the

Godfather blaring over loud speakers. The two young hostesses, given the pointless job of escorting diners to their seats at a pre-paid buffet breakfast, were dressed in full-length black evening gowns with red fur stoles.

While in Beijing, we had lunch at a large restaurant inside an indoor garden with a glass roof. The restaurant, which looked like a candidate for HGTV *Extreme Decorators China Edition*, was filled with live trees, vines, and pots of enormous cacti. There were dozens of fountains in all shapes and sizes. Various generic dragon statues, token Lucky Cat figurines with bobbing paws, and inevitable frogs with coins in their mouths were everywhere we looked. The glass ceiling was covered with red lanterns and large silk banners, blocking any view of the sky.

The last thing I expected to find in a restaurant near the Great Wall was a décor combination of standard Chinese interior design concepts and the desert foliage reminiscent of my childhood in northern New Mexico. It was a rather bizarre mix of retirement-home wicker furniture, Chinese take-out restaurant décor, and giant Saguaro cacti.

The atmosphere was chaotic, the noise level was intense, but the food was great.

According to Laura, "Chinese chefs believe a loud restaurant indicates that people are having fun and talking about the good food. If restaurants in China put up no smoking signs, they wouldn't have any customers because socializing in China—in addition to being noisy—revolves around tea, alcohol, and cigarettes."

We had a romantic dinner of Beijing's famed Peking roast duck at one of the original imperial duck restaurants. The grand affair included duck wings, cucumber in vinegar, duck feet with bamboo, mushroom soup, and roast duck breast with pancakes.

Chris found the duck feet most appetizing. After hesitantly trying a single bite of duck, which in my opinion tasted like roasted silly putty, I stuck with the mushroom soup. While the restaurant was stunningly elegant, the elaborate meal seemed wasted on our simple tastes. Still, we could have fared worse.

They say that Chinese eat anything with four legs, except tables; anything with two legs, except humans; anything that flies, except airplanes; and anything that swims, except submarines. It must be true since there are more than five thousand different dishes in China. As testament, the Guolizhuang Restaurant in Beijing served all types of animal penises, including yak, donkey, and deer, not to mention sheep gonads. Many Chinese people believe eating animal penises does wonders for women's skin. They also believe it increases male potency. (Chris still passed.)

One acclaimed fertility-boosting Asian delicacy I hoped to try while in China was bird's nest soup. Eating a swiftlet bird's nest is thought to get the baby-making juices flowing and increase the mood for love. The birds make the nests solely with their saliva—no twigs, branches, or leaves. The nests are soaked overnight and mixed with chicken stock, and, I assume, a ton of salt. Sadly, the very rare and highly coveted dish runs in the same circles with caviar, truffles, and Wagyu steak—way beyond our price range.

According to Laura, the Chinese believe there are three places for good food: Beijing, Shanghai, and Guangzhou. However, many Chinese cities have trademark dishes: in Beijing it is roast duck; Yangshuo has fried rice; Suzhou is known for shellfish; Guangzhou is known for suckling pig (and stewed dog and cat meat) and people love Shanghai's hairy crabs.

She added, "Rice is the main staple in the south of China, but in the north, we like our noodles."

Beijing was truly a feast for the taste buds!

It also provided fodder for reflection and thought. Tiananmen Square borders the Forbidden City, just on the other side of the Gate of Heavenly Peace, now known as the Tiananmen Tower. The tower, which served as a gatehouse in the Ming and Qing dynasties, has become a symbol of modern China after Mao Zedong stood atop the tower and proclaimed the founding of the People's Republic of China on October 1, 1949. His enormous portrait, flanked by the words "Long Live the People's Republic of China" and "Long Live the Great Unity of the World's Peoples," hangs on the tower.

At the entrance to the square was a rather confusing sign with simple stick figure images, crossed out with red circles. The sign indicated no motorized traffic, dogs, littering, flower picking, fires, or guns. It also seemed to forbid ice skating, falling leaves, and sitting on a bench with your legs crossed. While the simple images were easily identifiable in any language, the last three rules—and a few others—left us guessing.

Along with hordes of tourists and teams of soldiers, the square was inundated with vendors hawking copies of the *Quotations from Chairman Mao Tse-tung*, otherwise known as the Little Red Book. First published in 1964, some sources claim 6.5 billion copies of the notorious book of political rhetoric have been distributed. During the Cultural Revolution, every Chinese citizen was unofficially required to own, read, and carry the book at all times or risk punishment at the hands of brainwashed and deadly teen soldiers known as the Red Guard. During this dark time, Mao waged war on ancient Chinese culture and thought by burning books, ruining musical instruments, and destroying countless works of art. In addition, he declared himself the one God and thereby attacked China's many sacred centers for religion.

I was very moved by a giant memorial with incredibly realistic statues of laborers, soldiers, farmers, and scholars working together as one. The scholar proudly held a book up in the air, while a farmer lifted a bunch of wheat over her head, and a solider held his gun across his chest. The statue was beautiful and deeply symbolic, with the imagery of all the different types of people who together make a nation thrive. The dichotomy between the statue celebrating the individual at the site historically associated with government control and oppression of citizens was profound.

Tiananmen Square didn't offer much in the way of beautiful or natural scenery but visiting the seat of communism in China left an impression; the square's tumultuous history and the aftermath of tragedy still lingered in the air.

From April to June of 1989, students led demonstrations throughout the country over rapid economic growth, inflation, corruption and social change in post-Mao China. The students called for democracy, greater accountability, and freedom of press and speech. At the height of the protests, roughly a million people gathered in Tiananmen Square. The protests were forcibly suppressed after the government declared martial law on May 20 and mobilized three hundred thousand troops in Beijing. Troops with machine guns and tanks killed hundreds of demonstrators, during what became known as the June Fourth Incident in China, and the Tiananmen Square Massacre throughout the rest of the world. The exact number of protestors killed has been widely debated and heavily censored.

I became rather emotional as I stopped to think about how far the communist government in China could reach into the lives of the people. While China's "One Child" population control policy had given us hope for a family, it had also torn apart thousands of Chinese families. Many parents were forced to give up children or have abortions, and women were required to implant contraceptive intrauterine devices (IUDs) after one child and undergo sterilization by tubal ligation after two children. From 1980 to 2014, 324 million Chinese women were fitted with IUDs and 108 million were sterilized. It's estimated the One Child Policy had prevented 400 million births.

China's family planning program began in 1979 and restricted the Han people, the largest Chinese ethnic group at 93 percent of the population, to having only one child per couple. The policy allowed exceptions for smaller ethnic minority groups only, and strict fines were imposed on all others. By 2007, 36 percent of the population was held to a strict one-child policy, while 56 percent of the population was allowed two children, but only if the first child was a girl.

While my infertility issues were devastating, they were between me and Mother Nature, not imposed upon me by my government. As eager as I was to adopt a little girl from China, my excitement was somewhat tainted with guilt and sadness for the family that wasn't given a choice. All I could do to relieve my conscience was study China's history, culture, and language so that I could share it with my adopted child. I was determined to surround her with her culture and always respect her heritage.

On a lighter note, Tiananmen Square is *the* place to fly a kite in Beijing, if not the whole of China. There is nothing more pleasant and joyous than watching small children and entire families fly exotic, colorful and playful kites together. Throughout our time in China, there were several breezy spring days when kites filled the air and it was truly uplifting.

While there are many different tales relating to the invention of kites, almost all origin stories come from China. One lovely legend tells of a rice farmer working his fields in a traditional bamboo hat. A gust of wind stole his hat, and as he ran to catch it, holding on to the hat's strings, he inadvertently discovered the joy of kite flying.

The Chinese believe that kite flying is good for the health because flying a *fengzheng* in spring expels excess heat and strengthens immunity. Throughout China's history, kites have been used to drop propaganda leaflets, blow up enemy camps, and catch fish. Many cities in China are known for their own style of kite. In the city of Weifang, long, multi-layered dragons are popular, and it holds a huge kite festival each spring.

While enjoying the spring day in Tiananmen Square I couldn't help but laugh as a giant, red squid kite lifted a little boy right off the ground. His father chased him while his grandparents hollered and clapped. But the highlight of my visit to that famous square was witnessing a young woman, dressed in business attire and high heels, casually "walking" a large brown and white guinea pig attached to a pink, sequined leather halter and leash. The best part was that from her nonchalant attitude, as she stood in one spot for a few moments chatting on her cell phone, it appeared to be her normal coffee break routine. As for the guinea pig, it appeared to be on strike.

As we were finding day-to-day life in China to be very alien to us, I was reminded of how my disjointed childhood and my husband's traditional upbringing couldn't have been more different. Our childhood stories are vastly dissimilar from each other even though we were both raised in the same country, speaking the same language, and surrounded by similar cultures (although some would say the East Coast and West Coast of the United States might as well be different countries.)

Chris was raised in a small town in Maryland with a stable, middle-class family. His parents worked multiple jobs at all hours to provide for him and his younger sister. While his parents may have always been busy working, he was well cared for and got to hang out in some interesting places, including the video arcade parlor and the hair salon his mother owned in addition to an accounting business. Chris experimented with dreadlocks, platinum blonde hair color, and a perm (that made him look like Michael Hutchence from INXS). Plus, he was given lots of freedom to explore the beaches, marshes, and informal skateboard/BMX parks of southern Maryland (and got into a fair amount of trouble from what I understand).

Chris' parents taught him a strong work ethic. His father was an electronics technician for the Navy and taught Chris how to fix just about everything—and how to figure out how to fix just about anything else. He longed to teach the many skills his father taught him to his own children someday.

I fell in love with Chris because he's intelligent, responsible, faithful, kind, and more. Despite my trust issues and emotional baggage, I knew I could depend on Chris, and I was right—he has never let me down. I knew he would make a great husband and father. I knew that he would always provide for us, not just monetarily but by being generous with his time and affection—which I learned early in life is the most precious gift of all.

As we wandered the streets of Beijing together each night, I greatly appreciated the fact that we travel so well together. We both enjoy meeting new people, trying exotic foods, soaking up culture, learning local history, and seeking out every possible adventure.

However, we quickly grew tired of attempting to haggle with street vendors to buy souvenirs and trying to decipher drink menus at local nightclubs. In China, one bargains for almost everything, and for the Chinese, bargaining is an unofficial sport, at which they reign supreme. Purchases are often made after several rounds of haggling, from the first price (given to unsuspecting foreigners) down to the special price ("only for you"), and if you're very patient and crafty, the elusive China price.

For foreigners, the chosen mode of communication when negotiating with salespeople is a calculator. The proceedings begin with pointing to the desired object, whereupon the vendor will hand over a calculator with a starting figure. Then, if you're feeling brave enough for battle, you enter your counter offer—and the games begin.

While a Chinese phrase book may help you speak with taxi drivers in basic pinyin (the official romanization system for Standard Chinese in mainland China), no dictionary or phrase book will help you negotiate with street vendors, decipher Chinese characters on street signs, or read menu options at a locals only restaurant. Therefore, without the help of pictures, translations, or a guide, you may end up spending a small fortune on fake jade or accidentally ordering plates of tuna eyeballs, chicken testicles, or a whole roasted pigeon.

As we walked hand in hand, restaurateurs tried to drag us into their dining establishments and several young people followed us claiming to want to practice English. Thankfully, Laura had warned us of a common teahouse scam where tourists are invited over for a cup of tea and conversation, then charged a ridiculous fee.

Navigating the busy sidewalks of Beijing was daunting, and crossing major intersections made me feel akin to the frog with a death wish, who dodged a variety of vehicles and logs, in the 1980s video game Frogger. So we ended up spending many relaxing evenings enjoying local theater.

It would have been a shame to visit Beijing without experiencing the legendary Peking Opera, even though the story line was completely indecipherable. The ancient form of Chinese opera arose in the late eighteenth century and combines music, singing, mime, dance, and acrobatics. While the actors' costumes were elaborate and colorful, the stage was sparse with no scenery, just a gold curtain.

Sun Wukong, or the Monkey King, stole the show with his crazy antics and added some humor to the incomprehensible tales. He appeared as a main character in the sixteenth-century, classic Chinese novel *Journey to the West*. In the story, he was born from a magic stone and acquired immortality after eating life-giving peaches and supernatural powers after practicing Taoism. It was rumored he could control the elements and pluck out his body hairs and transform them into other creatures, weapons, or clones of himself. He rebelled against heaven and was imprisoned under a mountain by Buddha, but later he accompanied a Buddhist monk, a pig and two people on a voyage West to retrieve Buddhist sutras. Upon meeting with evil monsters, the monkey fought them off with a magic staff. (On a sidenote, the lead female's voice was not of this world and could have easily driven any enemy to submission.)

The opera at the Liyuan Theater was a truly authentic Chinese experience. As an added bonus we were served tea by a man who poured the steaming hot beverage through a long-spouted tea pot, from behind his back, into tiny tea cups the size of overgrown thimbles.

On a whim, we also bought tickets to *Chun Yi: The Legend of Kung Fu* at the Red Theater, and I'm very glad we did because I loved every minute. *Chun Yi* tells the story of a poor boy on a journey to become a warrior monk. It was hauntingly beautiful, completely thrilling, and surprisingly funny. It was equal parts ballet recital, kung fu demonstration, magic show, musical revue, comedy routine, pyrotechnics display, and acrobatics spectacle that rivaled Cirque du Soleil. It was as if my favorite Stephen Chow movie, *Kung Fu Hustle*, sprang to life on stage (which would be totally awesome). I felt emotions I hadn't felt in months, if not years, as I smiled with joy, hollered with amazement, and laughed until tears streamed down my face.

I couldn't remember the last time I'd laughed until I snorted.

While in Beijing we took a day trip to visit the magnificent Summer Palace (Yíhéyuán). Within the main courtyard are two large statues of lions standing watch. In China, they are called *shí shī*, meaning stone lion. Westerners call them Foo Dogs, probably because they look like curly haired dogs, possibly a ferocious Golden Retriever or rabid Sheep Dog. I learned that Imperial Guardian Lion statues, not only defend palaces, temples, and homes in China, but are also symbols of dedicated, watchful parents.

Guardian lion statues are always in pairs for harmony and balanced yin and yang. The male lion sits on the right, with a ball under his paw, to represent protecting the world outside the home. The female lion sits on the left with her paw on a young lion, symbolizing protecting her cub and all things inside the home.

It's been said that, like lions, mothers will go to extreme lengths to protect their children. In the heat of the moment, mothers have been known to lift cars, take on tornados and stare down wild animals to keep their children safe.

This got me thinking about the stereotypical Asian tiger mom. These strict, demanding mothers are known to push their children to academic superiority, musical perfection, and athletic success—as well as nervous anxiety. I realized that due to my long and difficult journey to motherhood, I was likely to be a total tiger mom, or as Americans would say a helicopter mom. I could easily picture myself anxiously fussing over my children, worrying constantly about their safety and keeping them on a short leash, like a crazed, mother Foo Dog.

After being "welcomed" to the Summer Palace by a pair of enormous and intimidating Foo Dogs, we spent the better part of a day exploring the imperial palace of the former Qing Dynasty (1644-1912) on the outskirts of Beijing. The palatial retreat was lovely but crowded, which is truly telling since the vast ensemble of lakes, gardens, courts, pavilions, and halls covers 742 acres.

The Long Gallery (Changlang), at 2,388 feet, is the longest painted corridor in China, if not the world, and is widely regarded as the most important feature of the Summer Palace. The covered walkway runs east to west, linking all the attractions along Longevity Hill and provided an observation platform of Kunming Lake. Emperor Qianlong built the corridor in 1750 so his mother could take long walks regardless of weather. The pathway is decorated with fourteen thousand paintings of animals, flowers, figures, and landscapes. There are four pavilions along the corridor, one for each season. Oh, to be so lucky, as to have such a devoted and loving child.

On Longevity Hill, the Sea of Wisdom temple houses a large collection of Buddha statues. Laura told us that if you admire Buddha, you should give him a glittering gift that shines like his wisdom. I immediately rummaged in my backpack but the only shiny object I could find on short notice was a stick of gum, which I figured wasn't a gift worthy of Buddha, despite the shiny silver wrapper. I was happy when Laura very enthusiastically accepted my offer of exotic, American, chewing gum and gave her the whole pack.

The moat surrounding the Forbidden City connected to Kunming Lake, so the royal family could leisurely boat to the Summer Palace. These days, tourists can take a scenic ride around the lake on ornate, colorfully painted dragon boats complete with mini pagodas. We opted for a round paddle boat with a roof painted pastel pink with lime green polka dots that looked like a cupcake. We very slowly circled the Island of Spring Knowing, so named because rumor had it the island could predict the changing of seasons due to its many willow trees that are sensitive to weather and herald the spring.

Visiting the Temple of Heaven, the Forbidden City, and the Summer Palace was an incredible experience due to their formidable size, powerful history, and stunning beauty. But once I learned the magnitude of planning behind the deeply symbolic, architectural details of these ancient sites—including their layout and the importance of color, numerology, and even tiny animal roof guardians—I reached a place of reverence. It was truly humbling to visit a place with such ancient history and tradition, where even the smallest, most seemingly insignificant design feature had value and purpose.

Even the sidewalks surrounding China's ancient palaces and temples were symbolically adorned. Stone dragons often crawled up center medians and countless steps had clouds carved on their sides to represent ascension to heaven. As I visited age-old temples, prayed to foreign Gods, and climbed cloud-adorned stairs, I longed to believe I was getting closer to realizing my dream of becoming a mother, and my positive aura started to show. I felt lighter, as if my once heavy footsteps now fell softer upon the earth.

One of the things that interests me most about cultures from around the world is their mythology and superstitions. Europeans knock on wood, Indians avoid cutting their hair on Tuesdays, and Russians never whistle indoors. A German would never toast with water, the Dutch don't lend salt to their neighbors, and many Asian cultures believe it is bad luck to trim your nails after dark. Never walk backwards in Portugal and remember to enter rooms in Spain with your right foot to avoid misfortune. Growing up in the USA, I learned to never step on sidewalk cracks, for fear it might break my mother's back!

The traditional neighborhoods in old Beijing are made up of *hutongs*, alleyways formed by a deteriorating labyrinth of courtyard residences, which provided a fascinating glimpse into ancient China and its many traditions and superstitions. When the Mongols invaded Beijing during the thirteenth century, they found little water, so they "asked" the local people to build wells called *hu*. Therefore, *hutong* means "area by the well."

We toured the old neighborhoods in a rickshaw, a covered cart pulled by an old man riding an even older bicycle. While bumpy, it was authentic, and less nerve-wracking than a crazy Chinese taxi ride. According to Laura, the hutongs were formed by the lines of the *siheyuan*, traditional courtyard houses. Each *siheyuan* had a square interior courtyard, many of which featured a jar of golden-colored koi fish. The ancient Chinese believed water brought wealth to a family, but only moving water, so they added fish to make the water living and lucky. The locals also often planted tong trees in the center of their courtyards since the tree was thought to attract phoenix, which brought families luck with finding wives and having daughters. We already had a small koi pond, but I made a mental note to research whether tong trees could survive Colorado's high altitude.

Every house had a horizontal beam at the base of the front door and a spirit wall in the center of the entrance hall to block the path of evil spirits, since the ancient Chinese believed ghosts move only in straight lines and can't jump. While no one wants a wandering ghost in their home, I'm guessing moving day in ancient China was a bit of a challenge and involved bribing friends with lots of *baijiu* (China's take on vodka).

Beijing's oldest residential areas were planned based on social class; at the center was the Forbidden City, surrounded in concentric circles by the Inner City and Outer City. Citizens of higher social status were permitted to live closer to the center of the circles.

The front doors of many homes displayed "flower stones" to indicate social status. A square flower stone looked like a book and indicated the residence of a civil servant. A round flower stone looked like a drum used in battle and therefore marked the residence of a military official. The most flower stones per residence was four, which indicated the highest possible position and social rank.

While the intricate layout of Beijing's old neighborhoods and the deeply symbolic adornments of the time-worn houses were fascinating, I was saddened by the overwhelming presence of classism and importance of social rank in ancient China (and throughout the history of our world). For the already downtrodden lower class, their social status weighed on their shoulders (and doorsteps) with a constant reminder of their inferiority and lesser value within their own community. At least the ancient Chinese placed a high value on intelligence.

In age-old China, classism didn't stop at the front door. A family's social rank greatly affected marriage prospects in addition to neighborhood planning. "In former times, a matchmaker could simply look at families' front doors and determine a 'gate marriage' of two families with a similar status," Laura told us. According to Laura, complex betrothal negotiations often began at birth, followed by a match and engagement during grade school and a teenage wedding. Since Confucian filial piety was widely practiced, the promised couple obediently accepted their parents' choice of spouse, sight unseen, until their wedding day. The matchmaker kept a list with the names and ages of available brides, then would introduce potential grooms to the waiting bride's parents. Next, an auspicious date was chosen for a meeting to assess the future daughter-in-law's appearance, character, and financial standing.

"The bride's eight dispositions, taken from the year, month, day, and time of her birth, were sent to the groom's family," Laura said. "The characters were considered as unique as fingerprints. A tablet with the girl's eight dispositions was set upon the boy's ancestral altar for three days. If the days passed without bad fortune or protest from the ancestors, the match was considered good. Then, the boy's eight dispositions were given the same test."

As a child, I was fascinated by a needlepoint plaque in the hallway of my grandmother's home which stated: "Monday's child is fair of face. Tuesday's child is full of grace. Wednesday's child is full of woe. Thursday's child has far to go. Friday's child is loving and giving. Saturday's child works hard for his living. And the child that is born on the Sabbath day is bonny and blithe and good and gay."

I asked my mother on what day I was born and was terrified to learn that I was born on a Wednesday. I didn't fully understand what *woe* meant as a child but remember thinking it sounded bad, and as fate would have it, my life has been a little heavy on the woe.

I often sadly mulled over the fact that my future, adopted daughter might never know her eight dispositions, or exact birth date, time, location, parents, religion, culture, or other circumstances. She would be one of many lost daughters of China, disconnected from her heritage and culture both literally and figuratively. My daughter would likely come with missing pages to her story that she would never be able to write.

On the other hand, she would grow up free from potential, self-fulfilling prophecies; for instance, family legacies and tragedies or being born "full of woe." Are we happier in our ignorance or knowledge—trying to manipulate our fate or letting destiny run its course? Either way, I felt the weight of not being able to provide my future daughter with answers to her starting point to help her along her journey. Her past might forever remain dim, so I simply hoped to be her bright future.

On our last night in Beijing, Laura gave me a gift. It was a pen with green ink that smelled like apples. "For the lady that is always asking questions and writing about China," she told me with a smile, "who will one day become a mother to a Chinese baby."

3

SEX AND DA CITY

We left Beijing on a Thursday via a loud and raucous two-hour flight on Air China to Xi'an. The second the plane's wheels touched the ground, the Chinese passengers got out of their seats, opened the luggage compartments, and began removing their bags. The flight attendants had to force several passengers to sit back down, then raced around closing luggage compartments as the plane taxied down the runway.

As soon as we got to the gate, once again everyone was out of their seats, crowding the aisle, and rushing the door as if the plane were on fire. The Chinese appeared always to be in a hurry and had no qualms about pushing and shoving their way to their final destinations.

As we deplaned and headed into the airport, there were no smiling faces to greet us nor little welcome signs bearing our name. We quickly began to panic, and I dug through my backpack searching for the customer service number for the China Highlights Tour Agency. After twenty minutes, we were approached by a lovely, young Chinese woman. As it turned out, our new guide, Zhang Zhao (who used the Western name Cheryl), and driver, Mr. Gu, were at the wrong terminal. I wouldn't have cared if Cheryl was late because she had been shopping for shoes and Mr. Gu had been drinking beer and watching a football match. I was just so happy to hear English and know that we weren't going to have to sleep at baggage claim.

During the drive to the hotel, Cheryl, whose Chinese name means rising sun, told us she has a boy's name because her father wanted a son. He had made a bet and named her before she was born. I felt sorry for Cheryl/Zhang Zhao and wondered how the Chinese people's favoritism of boys had affected her throughout her life.

Chinese law and tradition dictate that sons care for aging parents and are responsible for ancestor worship (not to mention superior help on a farm and perpetuation of the family name). Therefore, after the one-child policy was passed in 1979, many Chinese turned to sex-selective abortions and female infanticide to avoid serious fines. Orphanages throughout China began to overflow with "less desirable" baby girls, sky-rocketing the number of Western adoptions.

"Chinese parents believe beautiful children should be given an ugly name to keep balance," Cheryl told us. "They also think children shouldn't have too many good things. So to keep children from becoming spoiled, they give them bad nicknames."

I was curious and thought about asking if she was given a bad nickname by her parents but decided not to borrow trouble.

As we drove through Xi'an, we immediately noticed the striking contrast between old and new. Formerly known as Chang'an, Xi'an is one of the oldest cities in China, the oldest of four ancient capitals, and the imperial capital during thirteen dynasties. The former city center is surrounded by one of the oldest, largest, and best-preserved fortified city walls in the world.

Meanwhile, modern-day Xi'an is a bustling, neon metropolis with a trendy, upbeat vibe. The city is home to fifteen centers for higher education, including major universities, military academies and technical colleges. The streets were literally crawling with young students.

Xi'an, as well as all the other former capitals of China, has a morning bell tower and an evening drum tower. For hundreds of years, the towers served as clocks, informing residents of when the city wall gates were opening and closing and to warn citizens of danger. The bell tower was always located in the east and the drum tower in the west. The ancient towers still rise above the chaos of modern-day Xi'an, from the centers of deadly, four-lane, roundabouts teaming with traffic.

Our first night in Xi'an, we strolled the bustling streets, past crumbling buildings with grass growing in the cracks, while taking photos of giant, digital billboards alongside brightly lit ancient monuments. The energy coursing through the archaic veins of the venerable city was fresh and youthful. There were so many young people and so much activity on the streets, it felt like graduation day at the University of Central Florida, the largest public college in the USA with nearly fifty-six thousand students—but it was just a typical Thursday night in Xi'an.

We came upon a chic, red and gold sign with a pinup girl silhouette that read "Sex and da City" on a corner in front of an ultra-modern, stylish glass façade Starbucks. We felt a bit guilty buying tea, especially green tea, at a Starbucks in China, but it was quickly turning cold, my throat hurt, and we could order by way of pointing.

My best attempt to describe Xi'an is that of an ancient civilization, say Mesopotamia, that had a fling with the Las Vegas strip, which led to the birth of a college town, try Berkley, that somehow managed to stay true to its Chinese roots.

Xi'an was filled to the brim with young students and young love. Everywhere we looked we saw young people holding hands, snuggling on park benches, and kissing in dark corners; it was enough to make anyone giddy.

I was flooded with memories of my whirlwind romance with Chris.

Ours was a modern romance involving Match.com (back when Internet-based dating was a brand-new concept). My college roommate worked for the company and convinced me to be her dating guinea pig (for research purposes only; I never expected to find love). I spent several months dating nonstop, from wealthy entrepreneurs desperate for a wife to sexual adventurists looking for new orgy members. (I wasn't interested in either.) Eventually I met Chris, a computer geek with a shaved head, numerous tattoos, a monster Jeep, and a collection of Viking weapons. I was more than a little apprehensive but quickly learned he's a thinker, adventurer, and animal lover with a heart of gold.

We had been dating only nine months when Chris lost his job due to downsizing and decided it was the perfect opportunity to do some traveling. He spent three weeks backpacking through Eastern Europe before I met him in Greece. Chris proposed the night I arrived in Athens.

Perhaps the timing could have been better. After all, in the twenty-four hours before he proposed, Chris had gotten stuck in Turkey due to a boat strike, been waylaid on the island of Kos, arrived in Athens early, and got only a few hours' sleep beneath a table in the hotel restaurant (since the hotel was full).

Needless to say, he was exhausted and nervous.

We had dinner at a charming restaurant with seating in a fragrant, flower-filled courtyard with a fountain. Chris was about to pop the question, when a loud, chain-smoking, Greek couple bypassed numerous empty tables to sit right next to us and ruined the romance. We had drinks at a rooftop bar with views of the Acropolis, which was lit up at night and simply enchanting. Then the band started to play, and a group of very drunk Greek ladies began to dance and insisted I join them. By the time we left to go back to our hotel, Chris was a complete wreck. We cut through an ally in the red-light district of Athens that smelled of piss. Finally alone, Chris stopped and told me to close my eyes and hold out my hand. He placed a diamond solitaire in my palm.

When I opened my eyes and saw the diamond ring, at first, I thought it was a fake, purchased as a joke from a local street vendor.

One look at Chris' anxious face and I quickly realized my mistake. While I wasn't quite ready for marriage, due to some serious trust issues, I knew enough to realize that Chris was worth hanging on to. I tentatively accepted his proposal and we began discussing wedding plans and our future amid a gathering of stray cats. We agreed to move in together, so I could observe Chris after a night at the bars, a bad day at work, and at all hours of the day and night (and so we could save on rent). Thankfully, during the year we shared a townhome in Boulder, I fell completely in love with Chris (just in time for the wedding!)

When it comes to our Greek engagement, friends and family agree that the most memorable story is how my engagement ring traveled to Greece.

Since Chris had been backpacking throughout Eastern Europe and staying in youth hostels before I met him in Greece, he couldn't safely carry my engagement ring in his pack. Therefore, before he left the States, he made arrangements for the ring to be mailed directly to our hotel in Athens. However, the FedEx agent Chris dealt with was not aware of the company policy on shipping high value items, and the diamond solitaire was returned to sender!

At the time, Chris was renting an old carriage house in Boulder on "The Hill," a neighborhood adjacent to the University of Colorado and crawling with college students. Chris' place was right next to a fraternity house, and the ring was left on his doorstep—with a bright yellow note explaining that FedEx could not insure or ship valuable jewelry!

Chris learned of the shipping debacle while at an Internet café in Bodrum, Turkey, during the boat strike. He bought a calling card and rang his friend Kathy, in Colorado, in hopes that she could retrieve the ring from his doorstep, but she was in a business meeting. So, he called his best friend (and future best man), Chuck, in Maryland, who continued calling Kathy every half hour until he finally reached her (on the fifth try). As soon as she learned of the emergency, she left work early, drove a half hour to Boulder and rescued my ring from the doorstep (and neighboring frat boys).

The ring was safe, but in Colorado. That's when Chris launched phase two of a desperate plan. He convinced Kathy to spin a tall tale that her little sister was traveling through Europe and would be passing through Greece on her birthday. She called me at work the day before my departure and begged me to take a birthday gift to her little sister.

I was livid! First of all, I happened to know that Kathy's little sister was attractive. After being apart from my boyfriend for three weeks, the last thing I wanted to do was share my romantic reunion with Chris—with another woman. Second, I didn't want to have to rearrange my backpack, which was already bursting at the seams, hours before an international flight.

But I couldn't say no, so the morning of my flight, Kathy arrived at my office with a large box, wrapped in Happy Birthday paper and a giant bow. I angrily wedged the box into my backpack, with zero concern for the safety of its contents, and unknowingly couriered my own engagement ring to Greece.

If ours was a love affair destined for happiness, the same cannot be said every time Cupid's arrow hits its mark.

Our guide, Cheryl, told us of a legendary love affair gone wrong, when we visited Huaqing Hot Springs Palace, well known for the ill-fated romance between Emperor Xuanzong and his favorite concubine, Yang Guifei.

I must confess that I took the name Huaqing Hot Springs Palace literally. I arrived at the former winter retreat for emperors and their concubines with my swimsuit in tow, expecting a relaxing soak, only to discover that the Huaqing Palace had been vacant and dry for centuries. The only hot springs to be found was pumped through decorative, metal, lotus-shaped fountains. I guess I should have read the fine print in the tour company brochure.

Nevertheless, it was here, in the bone-dry Hot Springs Palace, that our guide told us about the consort Yang Guifei's legendary beauty—and also perhaps a bit more than we needed to know about her personal hygiene.

Born Yang Yuhuan, but best known as Yang Guifei, literally "Imperial Consort Yang," and one of the Four Beauties of ancient China, at the age of fourteen she married the Prince of Shou. However, the prince's father, Emperor Xuanzong became enamored with her and arranged for her to become a Taoist nun, to lessen criticism, before designating a new wife for his son and making her his concubine. Although he was rumored to have had three thousand concubines at his disposal, Emperor Xuanzong wanted only Yang Guifei.

The emperor had a penchant for spending an exorbitant amount of funds expanding the luxurious hot springs palace during the Tang Dynasty (618-907)—and he outdid himself when it came to pleasing Yang Guifei. He built numerous private pools including a roofless pool for star gazing, a lotus shaped pool for himself and a Chinese crabapple-shaped pool for his favorite concubine, Yang Guifei.

"During the Tang Dynasty, a full figure was considered more beautiful," Cheryl explained. "Lady Yang would sweat more, due to her plumpness, and had a bad odor, so she liked to bathe regularly. The emperor spent lots of money to have the floor of her personal pool lined with jade."

The emperor became completely obsessed with Yang Guifei, lavishing expensive gifts on her and her family, neglecting his duties as emperor and ignoring the plight of his people. It wasn't long before the masses began to rebel and Yang Guifei was accused of being an evil temptress.

Ultimately, she was likely murdered at the age of thirty-seven. Different accounts claim she was strangled by the emperor's personal attendant, banished or possibly escaped to Japan, or hung from a tree in the palace courtyard. All that remained was a tomb of her lavish clothes.

As I gazed upon the beautiful, white marble statue of Yang Guifei in the courtyard, I reflected on the challenging plight of women throughout history. I considered how Yang Guifei's beauty both benefited her and ultimately destroyed her. I thought about how so many women throughout the whole of history have been forced to use their bodies to provide pleasure, income, sustenance, and children.

It wasn't the first or last time I pondered my current state of infertility and how it might have affected me throughout history. Less than a century ago, my inability to conceive a child would easily have been grounds for divorce. I might have been thrown out on the streets and destined to a life of spinsterhood—and being labeled as barren. Even today, many couples dealing with infertility fall prey to adultery and divorce. My husband is his parents' only son and the last male to bear his surname. Though Chris and his family never put any pressure on me, I always felt responsible for helping to carry on the family name.

As much pain as my years of infertility caused me, at least my husband stood by me through miscarriages, fertility treatments, and adoption plans. This was one of many times that self-reflection would leave me feeling ashamed, faulty, and apprehensive during my battle with infertility.

Time marches on, and as I looked toward the hills surrounding the palace, I could barely make out a modern gondola ride slowly snaking up the side of Mount Li.

Only in China can six or seven cars, in a desperate effort to be the leader, span the width of a four-lane highway, together with bicycles and mopeds, while drivers communicate via an angry symphony of blaring car horns. I can guarantee that a taxi ride on the super highways of China is more thrilling than any gravity-defying, high-speed roller coaster in the world.

Our driver in Xi'an, Gu Chao, smoked a never-ending supply of cigarettes, drove incredibly fast and violently, and introduced us to a new form of swearing via a car horn all while listening to the gentle, folk music of John Denver. We got a good laugh out of listening to "Thank God I'm a Country Boy" as we careened, at top speed through the narrow streets of old Xi'an. Gu Chao spoke no English but was determined to sing along. It sounded something like "Tink Gwad I Tuntwee Bay." At his insistence, Cheryl informed us that he shared the same name as a famous Chinese Super League footballer, a fact that she was required to share with all taxi fares.

Gu Chao wasn't the only one who shared a name with his fellow countrymen; several thousand Chinese citizens share the exact same name, and it causes a lot of problems. In China, names begin with the surname followed by the given name. Friends and colleagues often address each other by their surname, not their given name. In the case of the most common surname Wang, an elder member might be referred to as Lao Wang or Old Wang, while a child might be nicknamed Xiao Wang or Young Wang.

Roughly 83 percent of China's 1.5 billion residents share *lao baixing* or "old hundred surnames." The name Wang is shared by some 93 million people, while 92 million citizens share the name Li and 88 million people go by Zhang. More than one hundred thousand Chinese citizens share the full name Wang Tao. In Beijing alone, there are more than five thousand people named Zhang Li.

In 2014, in hopes of reducing the high number of erroneous arrests, bank account errors, and surgical mishaps due to name confusion, the Chinese government began to allow parents the option of combining their surnames when naming their children.

Even though the name was unoriginal and widely used, we loved the simple name Mei (pronounced May) for our little girl. The name has not one but two lovely meanings: plum blossom when spelled Méi and beautiful when spelled Měi. We liked the idea of Dong-Méi, which translates to "winter plum blossom," as our daughter would be growing up in the Rocky Mountains. However, we couldn't get past the connection with Long Duk Dong from the eighties movie *Sixteen Candles*. Traditionally, Mei-Mei was a cute nickname for a little sister or pretty young girl, but for some odd reason became the nickname Chinese fans used for the American singer Taylor Swift. So, we settled on simple, beautiful Mei.

4

"SEVEN HAPPINESSES"

As I traveled through China, I began to wonder if I should learn more about some of the religions practiced in the Celestial Empire, including Buddhism, Taoism, and Confucianism in preparation for raising a Chinese orphan. Of all the world religions, I have always been most fascinated by, and naturally drawn towards, the tenets of Buddhism.

According to Cheryl, Buddhism strives for harmony of the mind, Taoism aims for harmony with nature, and Confucianism seeks harmony with society. All worthy goals, but at that point in my life, after my long struggle with infertility had shattered my emotions, more than anything I needed some harmony of the mind and spirit.

My crash course in Buddhism began at the Da Ci'en Temple. Centuries ago, the Buddhist monks of the Da Ci'en Temple were starving and prayed for food, whereupon a large, wild goose fell from the heavens. Instead of eating the goose, the monks buried it to show their gratitude. Another version of the tale claims the goose fell from the sky to teach the monks to be more pious, whereupon they stopped eating meat. Either way, Big Wild Goose is a fitting name for the temple's legendary pagoda.

Cheryl told us of an ancient Chinese phrase *chén yú, luò yàn*, which literally means "sink fish, drop goose," but is an expression to describe a woman who is stunning enough to sink fish and make geese drop from the sky.

Built in 652 during the Tang dynasty, when simple was considered beautiful, the pagoda originally had five stories, but two more stories were added to represent the seven stages of enlightenment in Buddhism. The temple was built to house the many Buddhist treasures, brought back from India by the monk Xuanzang. The book *Journey to the West*, about his seventeen-year-long pilgrimage, is of great importance to Chinese scholars and Buddhists (and includes the fabled Monkey King from the Peking Opera).

The lovely but stifling scent of incense and candle wax filled the air. Several giant, ornate, metal incense burners released constant streams of scented smoke while worshippers lit tall red candles and added them to huge racks in front of the temples. Many Chinese believed that smoke helped raise their prayers to the heavens. Sadly, most temples in China have moved to electric candles due to the high rate of pollution throughout the country.

Cheryl told us that her parents brought her to the Da Ci'en Temple when she was only two, and one of the monks gave her an orange from the table of offerings for Buddha. Believing the orange to be a token of good luck, her parents invited the entire extended family over to partake in the single auspicious orange.

The Great Hall of the Buddha housed an incarnation of the founder of Buddhism and Prince of India, Shakyamuni. A mural carved from a variety of colored gems and stones conveyed his incredible life story.

In a nutshell, Shakyamuni was born when his mother dreamt of a white elephant, and a baby sprang from her ribs. The child could immediately walk and took seven steps atop lotus buds. He pointed one finger toward heaven and one toward earth as he spoke to the people. Distraught that he couldn't solve the people's problems and hoping for an epiphany, he lived alone in a cave for five years, becoming sick from near starvation. Immediately upon his departure, he saw an apple, took a bite and created Buddhism, since Buddhism should be like the apple and provide comfort and relief. Three women representing joy, love, and lust tried to tempt him, but he resisted. At the age of eighty, he died and reached Nirvana, a place of neither life nor death, just peace.

This miraculous story of Shakyamuni made Scientology sound completely plausible despite being created by a science fiction author who believes in an evil alien named Xenu and that humans evolved from clams.

During times of great hardship and sadness, many people throughout the world turn to their faith for support and guidance. However, I was not raised with religion and had no real faith nor higher power to turn to during my struggle with infertility. One of the reasons I've never been very religious is because I observed my father "put on a show" while attending church on Easter and Christmas, the only two days a year I ever saw him pretend to be faithful. Each year at Lent, he gave up alcohol for six weeks, only to return to drinking too much and too often. My only experience with church, outside of major holidays, was that of my parents occasionally taking advantage of the free daycare. Even to a kid, it felt like false devotion (and I was always embarrassed for not knowing the words to prayers and hymns). I was spiritually alone.

I first learned of Guan Yin, commonly known as the Goddess of Mercy, while visiting the Da Ci'en Temple. According to

Chinese folk legend, Guan Yin's mother was dying, and the only cure was her own daughter's body; so, she selflessly offered her eyes and hands. Buddha was touched by Guan Yin's sacrifice and granted her the powers of Buddha. It's said that those that practice Buddhism develop a third eye allowing them to see Guan Yin's one thousand helping hands. She is most beloved by women, who pray to her for food, a good marriage, and children.

Guan Yin's story caused me to reflect on the powerful love between me and my own mother. She was the one loyal and loving constant in my difficult tumultuous childhood. I longed to share a bond with a child as strong as my link to my mother and experience the profound love between a mother and her child.

Not being raised with religion, years of failed pregnancy attempts, multiple miscarriages and unanswered pleas for a child did not help to increase my faith in a benevolent higher power. I had many tearful "Are you there, God, it's me Nina," episodes. I questioned whether or not a god or gods existed, and if so if they would listen to a fledgling believer? I wondered why they allowed me to suffer? I worried if I had caused some offense or committed some sin to deserve this hell. I wanted to believe and find comfort in religion but was timid and adrift in questions, fear, and doubt. I searched hopelessly for the root to my misery; was my infertility karmic, genetic, psychological, philosophical, environmental, hormonal, temporal? I questioned my family history, my life choices, my lifestyle and diet, my lack of religion. I searched tirelessly for answers and never found any . . . until China began to speak to me. It was as if China woke me from an agony-induced stupor and turned my humanity switch back on.

During my quest for motherhood, while I didn't practice any religion, I remained open-minded and welcomed guidance; therefore, I felt instantly drawn to Guan Yin. I believed her to be the perfect deity to hear my appeal for a baby. I wrote my wish on a wooden plaque with a red string attached and hung it on a hook alongside hundreds of other prayers next to a statue of Guan Yin. The statue sat in a beautiful garden filled with spring flowers just starting to bloom and chickens with fancy mohawk hairdos wandering around tiny, red velvet stools for praying.

Along with a prayer card and red candle, I purchased a delicate, pink candle shaped like a lotus flower sitting atop a green plastic pedestal stem and covered with gold sparkles. Buddhists believe the lotus to be a symbol of purity of mind, body, and speech since the flower is rooted in muddy water but rises above attachment and desire to bloom on the surface, having reached enlightenment. Buddha is often shown sitting atop a lotus bud to symbolize his having reached the pinnacle of enlightenment. The lotus became a symbol for my motherhood mantra: To rise above the darkness of infertility to blossom in the light as a mother . . . someway, somehow, someday.

For good measure, I decided to begin focusing my mind on elephants at bedtime in hopes that dreams of magical white elephants might prompt the miraculous conception of a divine baby.

One afternoon we took a relaxing two-hour, bike ride along the top of the old city wall, on equally ancient and rusty rented bicycles. We slowly meandered along, taking our time and stopping to view the scenery, both old and new. For once we were not on a tight schedule, without a guide and able to enjoy the many faces of Xi'an.

The ancient military defense system was forty feet tall and forty to forty-six feet wide at the top and fifty to fifty-six feet thick at the bottom. The wall was eight and a half miles long, formed a rectangle, and once had a deep moat around it. There was a rampart with a sentry tower every four hundred feet, covering roughly the range of an arrow from one tower to the next, for a grand total of ninety-eight ramparts.

The wall was lined with ornate, wrought-iron flagpoles flying small red and yellow flags. At the top of the flagpoles, delicate, metal swirls that looked like dragons or possibly phoenix with long tails, held strings of three, large red lanterns. A man in a bright blue jumpsuit swept the wall using a five-prong bamboo broom with giant ostrich feather plumes (dyed red, of course).

Like most cities in China, Xi'an is expanding and developing, a city under construction, a city of cranes. The skyline was dominated by cranes—small, medium, and large, every color of the rainbow, furiously destroying and creating day and night. There was a ceaseless clamor of jackhammers, wrecking balls, and crumbling cement, like the constant drone of department store Muzak during the holiday season.

The modern business district, filled with enormous shopping malls, glittering skyscrapers, and wide aven. es, was outside the ancient wall. Within the wall were slums filled with crumbling apartment complexes with sagging balconies and air-conditioning units precariously leaning off window ledges. Long forgotten, vacant dwellings with mostly broken windows were in various states of demise. Several buildings sat partially torn down and abandoned, like the demolition team went on a lunch break and never bothered to return and finish the job. There were empty lots filled with rubble, trash, and stray cats, plus miles upon miles of clothesline.

There was a heartbreaking contrast between modern, downtown Xi'an full of new development and vitality against the backdrop of the forgotten ancient city center within the wall which imparted a feeling of decay, loss, and sadness. Like Xi'an, I had built a wall around myself. On the exterior I looked happy and functioning, but inside I was broken and crumbling.

We asked Cheryl how she felt about her rapidly changing hometown. She simply sighed and shrugged her shoulders and then told us a story about two eighty-year-old women, one American and one Chinese. The Chinese woman said, "Now I can buy a house," while the American woman said, "Now I have finally finished paying for a house." The moral to this tale is "how long does the Chinese woman have to enjoy her house?" According to Cheryl, modern Chinese people have begun to borrow more money and acquire more debt—it's the American way.

When Chris and I got married and thought about starting a family, we upgraded from a townhome in the city to a cookie-cutter development in the suburbs—putting the proverbial cart before the horse. Now, we were trapped in a large bare nest surrounded by mini vans, baby strollers, and playgrounds on every corner—daily reminders that the house doesn't make the home.

One of my favorite memories of Xi'an is of an afternoon spent soaking up the sounds, sights, smells, tastes, colors and intoxicating, vibrant energy of the Muslim Quarter.

We enjoyed a leisurely stroll around the old Muslim neighborhoods of Xi'an, which dated back to when the city was the starting point of the famous Silk Road and many Muslims followed it to China to trade and start businesses. Xi'an became the first city in China to officially allow the practice of Islam and has remained home to a large Muslim community, mostly of the Hui minority.

The Great Mosque of Xi'an was built in 742 AD. It looked incredibly old and fragile. Grass was sprouting through cracks in the walls and growing along the crumbling eaves; it seemed the slightest breeze would reduce it to a pile of rubble and dust. It was rather remarkable to see an Islamic mosque with traditional Chinese peaked roofs instead of the typical white Islamic minarets. There was an abundance of antiquity, peace, and quiet reflection; meanwhile, the surrounding street markets were bursting with chaotic energy. Throughout the Muslim Quarter the calls to prayer could be heard over loud speakers.

The narrow lanes of the Muslim Quarter were tightly packed with Chinese pharmacies, sesame oil factories, and Halal permissible restaurants. There appeared to be at least one butcher shop on every block with large window displays of dangling heads, coiled loops of intestines, and tied bouquets of hoofs and tails. While I didn't have the stomach to venture inside, I could hear a cacophony of grinding, hacking, scissoring, chopping, beating, and sharpening, like a finely tuned orchestra of death.

Throughout the Muslim Quarter, row upon row of stalls displayed dried fruit, meat on sticks, and various nuts in bulk. Every type of tea imaginable was available in large rattan bowls, plastic bags, and ornate boxes and tins. Vendors sold silk fans, clothes, shoes, and scarves; small scrolls painted with landscape scenes and calligraphy; a wide variety of pottery and folk art; as well as a huge selection of knock-offs, cheap souvenirs, and other junk. Swarms of street merchants hawked a variety of lucky cat statuettes; low-quality terra-cotta warriors; cheap jade pendants and bracelets; kitschy Chairman Mao knick-knacks; and tiny, round, silk hats that looked like the Chinese version of a Jewish kippah. Upside-down umbrellas and bamboo bird cages hung from the rafters, and the sky was filled with strings of mini red lanterns, good luck talismans, and every type of kite in creation.

Women in colorful headscarves sold an array of spices—piles of earthy brown cinnamon, bright yellow saffron, rusty orange turmeric, creamy pale ginger, and lively red paprika— in huge metal bowls. Nothing was hermetically sealed under layers of plastic; it was all on display to be smelled, touched, and tasted (and susceptible to wandering cats, rampaging toddlers, or a gentle breeze).

Tourists and locals alike flocked to the Muslim Quarter for Halal snacks and regional delicacies including marinated meat in a baked bun, red bean cubes with Shaanxi spices, pita bread soaked in lamb soup, and Xi'an dumplings. Women baked scallion pancakes on makeshift ovens made from large barrels and prepared giant bowls of fried rice. I completely devoured a huge piece of flatbread straight off the burner with an image of Hamsa, or hand of Fatima, scorched onto one side.

It was a delightfully intoxicating mix of old and new, practical and souvenir, authentic and fake. An old woman not more than four feet tall sold beautiful handmade quilts and other textiles next to a young man in an LA Lakers jersey selling bootleg DVDs. As we walked past merchants, they hollered "Hello," "One Dollar," "Hello Lady," "Sunglasses," "Nice," "T-shirts," "You Like," "Hello!"

I was thrilled to buy some Shaanxi region folk art (the kind of locally made handiwork you won't find on Amazon). I bought three embroidered silk quilt squares from the tiny, old woman.

As I handed her a hundred yuan bill, she grabbed both my hands, squeezed them, and gave me a radiant, albeit toothless, smile.

During the nearly two years since starting our adoption process, I had begun a project for my future child based on the Chinese tradition of a One Hundred Wishes Quilt. While waiting for a baby to arrive, pregnant women in China often collected pieces of symbolic fabric from family members and close friends. Then they would weave together a quilt filled with the warm wishes of loved ones represented by a piece of Grandma's blanket, Auntie's wedding gown, and Grandfather's military uniform, for example.

My mother had already begun stitching together quilt squares donated by our family and friends. My half sisters contributed a bit of their grandmother's lace, a favorite T-shirt, and a soft flannel pillow case. Several cousins and friends donated pieces of beloved baby clothes and newborn maternity ward hats. The quilt also featured a souvenir shirt from our honeymoon in Costa Rica, Chris' cherished Outcrowd concert T-shirt and remnants of family heirloom quilts. I also created an album with the many letters from family and friends, which were included with the fabric donations, so my future daughter would be surrounded by welcoming images and words.

I told Cheryl about my project, and she informed me that I must buy a fabric piece embroidered with the Five Deadly Animals. In lieu of baby farm animals, choo choo trains, and pink elephants, the Chinese believe that surrounding a newborn baby with images of scorpions, snakes, spiders, centipedes, and lizards (or any other deadly creature an American mother would avoid) protect the child from harm. She added, "Chinese people believe all babies are perfect and evil spirits want to steal them. So, they

cut the top of a baby's finger—left for a boy and right for a girl—
to ensure this imperfection will keep them safe."

I was thrilled to find the perfect deadly animal fabric square
for my quilt but planned to alter my faithful following of Chinese
tradition when it came to cutting my future daughter's finger—
maybe just a paper cut.

My tiny, toothless friend was so charming I couldn't resist a
second, rather expensive purchase of an embroidered silk wall
hanging of One Hundred Lucky Babies. The narrow, two-foot-
long fabric featured one hundred Chinese children at play in a
rock garden, flying traditional Chinese kites, catching fish and
rowing boats along a river. My latest purchase elicited a full-on
hug and photograph with my new, Chinese bestie.

More than a million tourists, Chris and I included, flock
to Xi'an each year for a glimpse of the famed Terracotta Army
because there's nothing remotely like it anywhere else in the
world; it's beyond belief.

The first terra-cotta warrior was accidentally discovered in
1974 by a farmer digging a well. Little did Yang Zhifa know, he
had just discovered what has been called the Eighth Wonder of
the World and is now a UNESCO World Heritage Site.

An extensive excavation of the site revealed a full army of
terra-cotta soldiers in battle formation buried in a giant tomb
alongside Qin Shi Huang, the first emperor of China. The emperor
unified China in 221 BC, putting an end to the Warring States
Period when the country consisted of seven different kingdoms.
He standardized the writing system, currency, and measures and
is viewed as the father of the Great Wall.

Upon the emperor's death in 210 BC, he was buried together with statues of roughly 8,850 soldiers, 130 chariots with 520 horses, and 150 cavalry horses; a terra-cotta version of the emperor's full army, there to protect and serve him in the afterlife.

For more than thirty-eight years, starting when the first emperor was only thirteen years old, seven hundred thousand people worked to create his elaborate tomb and the warriors who guard it. Then, for two thousand years after the emperor's death, no one knew of the tomb, since allegedly everyone involved was killed to keep the secret. The skeletons of more than five hundred slain workers were discovered within the mausoleum, some of their arms were tied.

While the mausoleum was impressive, it was also intense, cold, and frankly a bit creepy! Seeing the burial chamber brought up the memory of my father teaching me to ride a bike at Fairmont Cemetery, one of the oldest (and therefore spookiest) cemeteries in downtown Denver. To him, it was a logical place to learn to ride a bike with its wide, flat roadways and little traffic. But to my young eyes, it was disturbing. I still check to see if I'm being followed by ghosts when I ride a bike.

The Terracotta Army was part of a larger necropolis that measured roughly thirty-eight miles wide. Pit one is the size of nearly three soccer fields and holds six thousand warriors. Pit two contains cavalry and infantry units, and pit three is the command post with high ranking officers. Apparently, pit four is filled with acrobats, dancers, and musicians, but it is closed to the public.

The terra-cotta figures are life sized and vary in height, uniforms, and hairstyles in accordance to rank. Allegedly, no two faces are alike, since they are thought to be exact replicas of the emperor's army. Almost all the original paint was gone, but the intricate facial details remained. Due to a peasant uprising the year after the emperor's death, most of the warriors' authentic weapons were looted or have long since rotted away.

"Five-star generals have long hair with double knots and three ribbons," Cheryl said. "Infantryman knot their hair on the right side and cavalryman have no knots in their hair and wear skirts for horse riding. The clay soldiers are hollow to house their souls."

While the mausoleum was one of a kind in its magnitude, artistic detail, and bizarre purpose, I had to wonder what sort of madness and paranoia could lead a ruler to create something as incredible yet also horrific as the terra-cotta warriors?

The gift shop was filled with hundreds of very expensive terra-cotta warriors, so we chose a single, small figurine of a kneeling warrior (high ranking, based on the hairdo). I was happy simply getting a photo of my head sticking out of a headless, terra-cotta soldier photo prop, like an ass-kicking warrior princess.

We saw the former farmer-turned local celebrity, Yang Zhifa, having a nap in a chair in the gift shop. He had just turned seventy-five. After the terra-cotta warriors were discovered beneath his fields, he sold his tiny plot of farmland, relocated to a new village called Qinyong or "Qin Warriors," and took a job signing autographs. We decided not to wake him.

Later that week we spent a pleasant hour at the former residence of the Gao family, which was one of the best-preserved traditional homes in Xi'an. The home, known as the Folk House, offered a rare and fascinating glimpse into traditional Chinese culture. It housed a museum, teahouse, shadow puppet and marionette theater, and an art studio with paper cutting demonstrations and painting lessons.

The mansion was the residence of Ming dynasty official Gao Yuesong and his family, seven generations of which became officials of the royal court from 1368 to 1644. The compound consisted of eighty-six rooms filled with authentic antiques, a private school, separate reception rooms for men and women, and several courtyards.

As I walked through the ancient Chinese mansion, I struggled to envision generations of Chinese children growing up there. The dysfunctional layout, closed-off rooms, and formal décor was anything but a welcoming environment for rambunctious toddlers. I had visions of young kids hanging from the interior balconies, swinging from the tasseled silk lanterns, and tripping over the ghost-busting door beams. I suppose any centuries-old home would look intimidating (and like a death trap) to modern parents obsessed with open floor plans; large fenced yards; and designated family, laundry, and mud rooms with lots of storage. (I'll admit, I'm an HGTV junkie.)

My own father's house was more museum than home. As a child, I didn't feel comfortable running around my house (god forbid I jumped on the beds). I would never put my feet on the couch (or leave behind the smallest mess), and I lived in fear of breaking my grandmother's china (or any other pretentious antiques). My room was decorated by a professional interior designer with antique dark walnut furniture, a peach and cream color palette, and framed prints from the Metropolitan Museum of Art. (My Duran Duran poster lived under the bed.)

In contrast, Chris and I had no fear of muddy footprints, crayon-smeared walls, and constant bedlam. Thanks to our two big dogs, our house was a perpetual furry disaster, and we were all for kids being kids, exploring their world and making regular messes.

Of all the insanely delicate, uncomfortable looking and non-kid-friendly pieces of furniture in the Gao mansion, the beds left the most lasting impression. The standout was a black lacquered, wooden, four-poster bed with wide window-like openings and a canopy top, all covered with red silk curtains. A matching red silk coverlet lay across the hard, thin mattress. The moon-shaped window openings were decorated with intricately carved wooden panels with flowers and landscapes. The entire box-like sleeping apparatus sat on legs several feet off the ground.

The uninviting sleeping contraption/torture device made me wonder if the design was based on a Chinese adaptation of the "Princess and the Pea" fairytale, having skipped the layers of soft mattresses and gone straight to the hard pea. By this point in my travels through China, I had already concluded that the Chinese prefer hard beds and would be completely perplexed by the American concept of pillow tops, goose feather duvets, and throw pillows.

As someone who suffers from regular bouts of insomnia, I've come to the conclusion that lack of sleep is the root of all evil, leading to depression, anxiety, a weak immune system (and no doubt infertility issues). Therefore, I take sleep quality very seriously. I eat dinner early, avoid caffeine (at least at night), take hot lavender-infused baths, listen to white noise, take valerian root supplements, and sleep in a ridiculously high-tech, Sleep Number bed. But to my surprise, while in China, I slept like a pampered (but crudely snoring) princess.

During our travels in China, I suffered from serious springtime allergies. My throat was raw, my nose dripped like a leaky faucet, and I had to sleep with my mouth wide open, leading to dry mouth that could rival the Gobi Desert. According to Chris, after several days of touring a highly polluted country in the springtime with a wife with severe allergies, asthma, and a deviated septum, every night felt like spooning Darth Vader.

My list of allergies is extensive: six trees, five grasses, eight weeds, two molds, penicillin, and all major narcotic pain meds. Combined with asthma and eczema, I'm considered atopic. Basically, my immune system is bat-shit crazy. For years, if I wasn't sitting in a fertility clinic waiting room, I was visiting with my pulmonologist or getting an allergy shot. After years of weekly allergy shots with mostly the same people, my fellow allergy sufferers became like a second family. The immunotherapy waiting room was always lively, with people bitching about pollen counts, commiserating with each other over allergy symptoms, and playing the "who has the greatest number of allergic triggers" game. I thought I had it bad, but one guy had forty-seven allergic triggers, giving him serious bragging rights and waiting-room cred.

Meanwhile, the reception area at the fertility clinic looked like a funeral parlor. Those suffering from infertility appeared half dead, avoided eye contact, and stared blankly at the floor or stealthily scoped the room, wondering about the age and condition of the other miserable patients. Sadly, striking up a conversation with a fellow female in the throes of infertility just didn't happen. We were all overwhelmed with stress, consumed with our own emotions, and didn't have the energy to willingly welcome more drama into our lives—even if some personal experiences may have helped us along our journey.

I'm sad to admit that while in the trenches of infertility treatments jealousy, insecurity, and fear run rampant. Few women can muster support or concern for others . . . until they have babies. Then, triumphant new mothers become champions for whatever drug, treatment, doctor, adoption agency, or bizarre fertility voodoo granted them motherhood. Suddenly, they become eager to share their story, lend a shoulder to cry on, and go above and beyond to support their fellow women still knee deep in shit.

Our room at the lovely Meihua Golden Tang Hotel was an oasis by day but became anything but relaxing at night, due to rice paper thin walls. We could hear our neighbor—who must have been a 350-pound sumo wrestler—snoring, coughing, and wheezing all night. If my allergies and asthma made me sound like Darth Vader, this guy sounded like a wookiee with sleep apnea, night terrors, and a major sinus infection.

We turned on a music television show in a desperate attempt to subdue the nervous breakdown–inducing, monotonous din but to no avail, so we resorted to reading. Thankfully, Chewie the sumo wrestler checked out after only one hellish night.

While staying in Xi'an, we received a call at our hotel room every night around 10:00 from a woman inquiring if we would like a massage. Aware of the alternative meaning of a massage in an Asian country, Chris and I had lots of fun dreaming up different massage options, with varying degrees of sexual innuendo. Some of our favorites included Crouching Dragon, Hidden Phoenix, Seven Happinesses, Pressure Luck, the Fortune Cookie, Double Golden Paradise, and, of course, the Happy Ending.

We did not, however curious, choose to partake in a massage, but did decide to get frisky.

After years of carefully timing intercourse to then stick with the gravitationally preferred, missionary position (per the recommendation of *Taking Charge of Your Fertility),* it was high time for some rowdy hotel sex. It was time we allowed ourselves to simply have fun, go with the flow, and express our love for each other—not just a desire for a child.

It was time to leave Xi'an. We left with full stomachs after lunch at an authentic noodle house, where we discovered our favorite Chinese dish: crispy fried green beans in garlic oil. It was the most enthusiastic I have ever seen my husband get about vegetables. In fifteen years of marriage, we continue to keep completely different (mostly carnivorous versus mainly vegetarian) diets, and it has been my responsibility to eat every one of his side salads, vegetable crudités, and dollops of guacamole. The man can't stand anything green but loves anything spicy.

The green beans made my lips tingle and tongue burn (and I grew up eating green chiles on everything). The dish was garnished with a beautiful flower carved out of some sort of root vegetable (perhaps a traditional Chinese breath mint, inadequate natural antacid, or attempt at a peace offering).

After lunch, we boarded a ninety-minute Air China flight for Guilin, traveling in a comfortable, modern jet with pictures of Olympic babies on its sides and tail. China hosted the Summer Olympics in 2008 and publicity for the event involved images of five childlike figures or *Fúwá*, which literally means "good-luck dolls."

Thanks to the in-flight magazine (which we kept as a souvenir), we learned all about the Olympic babies. The *Fúwá* included Beibei, a blue fish, representing Europe and aquatic sports and symbolizing water and prosperity; Huanhuan, the red Olympic flame, representing America and ball sports and symbolizing fire and passion; Yingying, the yellow Tibetan antelope, representing Asia and track and field and symbolizing earth and health; Nini, the green swallow, representing Oceania and gymnastics and symbolizing metal and good fortune; and finally, Jingjing, the panda bear, representing Africa and weightlifting and symbolizing wood and happiness. Together, the names form the sentence *Beijing huanying ni*, which means "Beijing welcomes you."

Sadly, the five mascots were also associated with tragedy. In the months leading up to the Olympics, coincidental similarities between the characters and several disastrous events led to talk of the Curse of the Fúwá and some Chinese calling the characters *Wuwa* or "witch dolls." Beibei, a Chinese sturgeon, was blamed for the 2008 South China Floods; Jingjing, the Panda for the Sichuan Earthquake; and Yingying, the Tibetan antelope, for unrest in Tibet.

However, good fortune came to China during the 2008 summer Olympics, when they dominated the medal rankings for the first time with the highest number of medals at one hundred, including forty-eight gold medals. The Chinese considered it extremely auspicious that the opening ceremony was scheduled to begin on August 8, 2008 at 8:08 p.m. This was because eight (*bā*) rhymes with the word for prosperity (*fā*).

The Olympic stadium in Beijing was called the Bird's Nest. Not only did it resemble a nest, but the Chinese people believed that a phoenix built the nest. Meanwhile, the National Centre for the Performing Arts is said to be shaped like an egg because the phoenix flew from her nest in the north to find food in the south and dropped an egg in the middle.

The five Fúwá were responsible for a rise in the birth rate in China. A headline in the *Beijing News* read "Olympic Babies Are Coming" after thousands more babies than usual were born in Beijing starting in 2008. Many of the children born during this Olympic baby boom were named after one of the adorable mascots.

During our flight to Guilin, Chris and I discussed the cute and sentimental notion of an Olympic baby name for our future daughter. However, Nini was too similar to Nina, and Beibei reminded us of BeBe from the adult animated show South Park. In the end, we weren't swayed from our love of the name Mei for our daughter to be . . . someday.

We were sorry to say goodbye to the vibrant, youthful energy of Xi'an. The city had helped us to laugh, live, and begin to love again. For a fabulous spell, we were young and full of puppy love, with nothing but blue skies ahead of us.

5

GREEN JADE HAIRPINS

After touring two of China's largest northern cities and viewing a staggering number of palaces, temples, and major historical sites, we were both overwhelmed and overstimulated. We were eager to slow down and revel in China's natural beauty, for which Guilin is famous.

While Guilin is roughly a quarter of the size of Beijing and half the size of Xi'an, at 4.7 million it is still a major city. It would be awhile yet before we saw some countryside, but even then, as we were soon to discover, "rural" is a relative term in China.

China's population of 1.5 billion, the largest of any country on earth, may simply be a statistic to the rest of the world, but to those living in China, it affects every aspect of life, including employment, commerce, the environment, standards of living, and social infrastructure. In a land that requires extreme population control measures, the crowded inhabitants seemed to have lost their sense of personal space, boundaries, and decorum.

I am not a city girl. I get unnerved and frustrated simply dealing with crowds at the mall, let alone navigating through a country as densely populated as China. I'm a Rocky Mountain girl; I need my sunshine, mountains, and wide-open spaces.

The city of Guilin, while still a bustling metropolis, was on the fringe of southern China's beautiful countryside and existed in the shadows of the lush, green hills of the northeast section of Guangxi province. The poet Han Yu described the hills of Guilin as green jade hairpins, while the poet Fan Chengda referred to them as jade bamboo shoots. Guilin was hauntingly beautiful, did not disappoint our need for some natural beauty and was a great starting point to our further exploration of China's famed Southern landscapes.

In China, it is said that a city without water is a city without vitality, but Guilin had plenty of both, thanks to the Two Rivers and Four Lakes scenic district, consisting of Rong, Shan, Gui, and Mulong lakes and their benefactors the Lijiang and Taohua rivers. Rong Hu was named after the eight hundred-year-old banyan tree on its shore, while Shan Hu was named for the Chinese fir and Gui Hu for the Osmanthus tree. The bodies of water began as humble city moats during the Tang dynasty but were reconstructed and expanded to create the city-wide waterway and scenic park system.

The gorgeous tree-lined lakes were bordered by several pavilions, rock gardens, statues and quiet sitting areas. Weeping willows dipped into the green water and bright pink flower bushes dotted their borders. Ornate, white marble moon bridges appeared to float above the narrow riverways while in the background, lush green hills rose suddenly out of the earth. Long, flat boats glided soundlessly through the perfectly still water.

The lakes were lined with adorable, cement pigs that doubled as benches. Numerous flat stones carved with Chinese characters bordered the trails and mushroom-shaped lamps hid in the bushes along the edges of the paths. A long, white marble, walkway zigzagged across the aquamarine water to a lovely, floating teahouse. The walkway's circuitous design protected against evil spirits who can walk only in straight lines.

It's no wonder the green hills, crystal waters, fantastic caves and spectacular rock formations of Guilin are often referred to as the finest under Heaven. We had arrived in a magical paradise; the stuff of ancient myths, folktales about unicorns, and legends of dragons.

I couldn't imagine a more perfect place for us to embrace our own happily ever after.

Since I married a man named Little, my bridal shower invitations read, "Nina's getting married and we're just a 'Little' happy for her." My half sisters hosted a brunch for me at our new townhome several months before our summer wedding. While Chris and his friends went snowshoeing, the party guests were busy designing wedding dresses out of toilet paper, playing the how well do you know the bride and groom game, and writing recipes for a happy marriage.

As I opened gifts, I was completely unaware that my comments were being recorded so that they could be taken out of context and related to the wedding night. "There's nothing in here," "Whatever this is, it is really heavy," "It's upside down," "Where's the...? Oh, there's the end," and "This isn't hokey; it's cute."

My sisters made party favors consisting of glass bud vases filled with Jordan almonds (for health, wealth, happiness, fertility, and longevity) topped with tiny drink umbrellas spray-painted periwinkle blue (to match the color of the bridesmaids' dresses). As an added touch, they wrote each guest's name on their umbrella and covered the umbrellas with sparkling tinsel.

It was a lovely, highly memorable (and slightly raunchy) affair (but perfectly tame in comparison to my bachelorette party!).

We had a small, garden wedding at a completely enchanting historic bed-and-breakfast. Not only was the century-old mansion surrounded by an English garden with a stunning view of the Rocky Mountains, it was located in Loveland, Colorado. We mailed our wedding invitations (a black and white photograph of two pears leaning against each other with the line "A Perfect Pair") on Valentine's Day from the local Loveland post office, just so they would receive a special love-themed stamp.

Since we got married over July Fourth weekend, we originally wanted to serve picnic food, but the chef was horrified so we switched to an upscale brunch for roughly one hundred. My college roommate (the one who convinced me to try Match.com) was my maid of honor and my bridesmaids consisted of my half sisters and a dear friend. Chris' groomsmen flew out from Maryland (and crashed in our basement, where they watched the movie *Old School* on repeat).

Our hippie officiant wore a tie-dyed silk robe and gave a lovely sermon based on Native American mythology. Our friends read a poem from *The Prophet* by Kahlil Gibran and an excerpt from *The Velveteen Rabbit*. In our new life together, Chris vowed whatever may come to never judge me, love me without question, encourage me to follow my dreams, comfort me, laugh with me, and cry with me (and to kiss my booboos and love my dog).

For wedding favors, we gave our guests postcards with photos of a variety of beautiful Colorado landscapes with handwritten love poems on the back and packets of Colorado wildflower seeds tied up with a ribbon and a single fresh daisy. Down the aisle and on every table were woven stick baskets filled with colorful wildflowers.

Even though we got married midday and it was over one hundred degrees, our guests still enjoyed local microbrews and mimosas, plus several hours of hard-core dancing. Instead of a limo, Chris and I drove away in his topless, monster Jeep, which his friends decorated with neon paint and streamers with cans.

Our wedding was perfect, and I wouldn't change a thing, except maybe my giant white tent of a dress. My advice to those getting married: never fall for the standard line to order your wedding dress two sizes larger. I'm convinced the boutiques and alteration businesses are in cahoots. I chose my dress based on the store sample that fit me like a glove, but even after three rounds of expensive alterations, my wedding dress fit like a silk burlap sack.

The day after our wedding, we were off to a honeymoon adventure in Costa Rica.

We arrived in San José in the middle of the night and left early the next morning for Tortuguero, an ecotourism mecca located on a sandbar along the Caribbean coast. We took a bus journey through fields of bananas, then a boat trip past caimans and coatimundis in order to reach the remote corner of Costa Rica known as the "Little Amazon." We hiked through a rain forest where local children caught poison dart frogs, so we could take a photo. Then they asked us for money. We visited a beach during an incredible lightning storm to look for hatching turtles. We went to a village of Nicaraguan refugees where we purchased local handicrafts. Then, we took a memorable road trip, attempting to navigate our rental car through a country with no street signs, only landmarks, to the base of the Arenal Volcano, where we zip-lined over a cloud forest and visited the heavenly Tabacon Hot Springs on a daily basis.

Next, we flew to the Golfo Dulce in a small airplane that landed on a dirt airstrip in the middle of a field. We stayed in our own treehouse bungalow where monkeys ran across the thatched roof and a pair of toucans lived in a tree just off the deck. We kayaked through bath-temperature water in the gulf, hiked to a waterfall, and lounged on the beach. I went for a "relaxing" massage in a thatched roof hut and spent the entire time fixated on a giant, hairy spider in a corner of the roof (this came after discovering an enormous snake curled upon the steps to the hotel pool).

Upon our return to San José, we stayed at an incredible coffee plantation resort with a waterfall bathtub and a honeymoon suite bedroom at the top of a tower with a spiral staircase. While vacationing in Costa Rica, we drank piña coladas every day (often out of carved pineapple glasses), ate exotic fresh fruit and gallo pinto (traditional dish of beans and rice), listened to the bellow of howler monkeys, and snuggled every night.

After our beautiful wedding and adventurous honeymoon, life was good, for a while. We sold our townhome in the city and bought a house in the suburbs. I completed graduate school and received a master's in elementary education. Chris took up running (and now has bad knees).

Then we tried to start a family.

And that's when all hell broke loose.

Four years later we ended up on the other side of the world nursing the wounds of our happily ever after gone awry.

If we were looking for distraction and healing, we began to find it in Guilin.

Nothing helps more to expand the soul, break down social barriers, bridge cultural gaps, and create new friendships than singing. And within five minutes of meeting our new guide in Guilin, that's exactly what we were doing—singing.

We took a day trip to the countryside surrounding Guilin with our new guide, Wei Mei Ping. Her name meant beautiful duckweed flower, but she chose to go by the English name of Claire. Together, we embarked on a two-hour journey by car to the Lóngshēng minority villages and the Dragon's Backbone Rice Terraces. Along the way, our very young and sweet new guide sang several Chinese folk songs for us.

Then Claire asked us to share an American song. I sang "Summertime," from the George Gershwin opera *Porgy and Bess*, which my mother sang to me as a child. Just for fun, I sang "Old MacDonald had a Farm," since I've always been amused by animal sounds in different languages. The delightfully inquisitive Claire already knew the song by heart, so we had great fun mooing, quacking, and meowing together on the way to Lóngshēng. In China, the dog goes *wāng wāng*, the duck goes *guā guā*, and the pig goes *hēng hēng*.

She taught us the Chinese lullaby, "*Liang zhi lao hu*," or "Two Tigers," sung to the tune of the French lullaby "*Frère Jacques*."

Two little tigers,
Two little tigers,
Run very fast,
Run very fast.
One has no eyes,
One has no tail.
Very strange,
Very strange.

Simple and catchy, but honestly a bit morbid! Then again, American children sing songs about plagues, prostitution, and burning witches at the stake—so no judgement here.

For the remainder of the road trip, Claire told us about her family. They moved to Guilin from the country for more education and employment opportunities. I'm guessing she was in her mid-twenties, and her father had only recently graduated from primary school. Her mother made bamboo beds. According to Claire, most people in Guilin worked from 9:00 a.m. to 6:00 p.m., with a two-hour lunch break, so they could return home to eat and rest. She said the Chinese believe in continuing to work throughout their senior years to keep their minds alert.

When I told Claire about our plans to adopt a Chinese orphan, she confided with sadness that several of her family members, neighbors, and friends had given up infants for adoption or been forced to abort their babies. She was happy one child would find a good home.

After our drive filled with music and laughter, we abandoned the car and hiked along a path through a series of villages populated by groups of Chinese minorities nestled amongst terraced rice fields. During the Mongolian-ruled Yuan Dynasty (1279-1368), many minority groups were forced to flee to the mountains. Being primarily an agricultural society, they needed to find a way to continue farming on the steep sides of the mountains. They ingeniously turned the mountains into farmland by creating terraced fields. To see the legendary terraced rice fields, we had to hike several miles into the foothills.

While the scenery all around Lóngsheng's minority villages was stunning, the area at the base of the hill leading up to the villages and rice terraces was commercialized and filled with tourists. The parking lot was packed with tour buses, taxis, and hordes of loitering shoppers. Business savvy entrepreneurs sold snacks, bottled water, and cold Coke, along with a variety of the standard, gaudy souvenirs. Children wandered around trying to sell postcards. There were a few permanent structures where actual residents sold more authentic handicrafts, namely pointed straw hats, colorful knit sweaters, and woven bags and purses.

Along the passageway, we saw a number of chaise lounge chairs that had been re-engineered into makeshift forms of transportation. The chairs were equipped with long, bamboo poles, fringed shade canopies, and colorful padded seats. Surprisingly petite men waited for lazy, wealthy tourists who wanted a ride up the mountain. The tourists would sit in the chair and two Chinese farmers would carry it by the poles jutting out of each end. Meanwhile, women transported tourists' luggage in large, straw baskets with shoulder straps. These Chinese farmers may have been small, but they were "strong like bull."

The path leading to the rice fields followed a river. Before long we found ourselves strolling through several small villages of large, wooden, thatched roof structures. These Zhuang-style homes were unlike any we had previously seen in China (and slightly reminiscent of Swiss chalets). Some were single-family homes and others were multifamily, apartment-style dwellings. Many of the homes were on stilts and precariously clung to the side of steep hills. Several long poles leaned against the structures at odd angles in a desperate attempt to keep the buildings from sliding down into the river. Apparently, the homes were built with no nails—not the safest building design for homes on the side of a cliff.

A network of narrow passageways and steep cobblestone stairs for pedestrian traffic, oxen, donkeys, and wandering chickens, snaked through the compact villages. There were no motorized vehicles. Red lanterns, colorful strings of laundry, and rows of yellow corn hanging from their husks filled the sky above where we walked. These villages truly defied the laws of gravity and rural quaintness and seemed like a very pleasant place to grow up, far from the chaos, noise, and negativity of our modern world.

There are a total of fifty-five different ethnic minority groups living throughout China. The rice farmers living in the Lóngsheng villages are members of the Yao, Zhuang, Miao, and Dong minority groups. The different minority groups living in Lóngsheng retain their own customs and languages but live in harmony alongside each other.

In Huangluo Yao Village, the women often wear embroidered costumes and heavy silver earrings but are best known for their long hair. According to Claire, Yao women hold the Guinness World Record for the longest hair. The women cut their hair only once, at the age of eighteen, then keep their long hair wrapped up in a bun.

"Their favorite color is red, therefore the locals call them Red Yao," Claire said.

As far as I could tell, everyone's favorite color in China is red. Red is the color of the flag of China, the color associated with happiness, and the official color of all festivals and weddings. Since it is the color of blood, red is associated with life in China. On the other hand, I associated red with the loss of life and regular reminders of the lack of new life, each and every month.

In Ping'an Zhuang Village, most women wear white shirts, black pants, and brightly colored head scarves. While the village was remote and inaccessible by car, it still managed to have a population of seven thousand and numerous hotels, restaurants, and shops—proving that even rural, farm towns in China were huge by most of the world's standards.

The villages were a truly unique, living museum of China's ethnic minority groups and a fascinating look at farm life in rural China; while the Dragon's Backbone rice terraces were an incredible feat of engineering and intriguing glimpse into China's long-standing rice industry. Plus, the day trip gave us an escape from crowded cities and offered us stunning scenery, fresh air, and wide-open views (but only because we were willing to hike above and beyond the mass of tourists).

The hills were layered with narrow tiered strips of farmland. The terraced rice fields blanketed entire mountains from base to peak. It was said, "where there is soil, there is a terrace." The rice terraces coiled around an area of roughly 16,000 acres and spanned an altitude from 980 to 2,600 feet.

We visited in spring, when the terraces were filled with water and the reflection off the water looked like rivers of silver in the mist. According to Claire, since the fields are dependent on rainwater and there is no irrigation system, they are called sky watering fields. The terraces are filled with water in spring, green shoots in summer, layers of rice in fall, and snow in the winter.

"Locals say the fields look like a twisting dragon in spring, green waves in summer, a golden beach in autumn, and a soaring silver dragon in winter," Claire told us. "The tiered rice fields look like a dragon's scales and the tops of the terraced mountains look like a dragon's backbone, so the fields got the name Dragon's Backbone (or Long Ji)."

Individual sections of the tiered fields are owned by different families, and entire families—from toddlers to mothers with babies on their backs to frail but determined seniors— work the fields together. In June, the rice buds are transplanted, and in October, the rice is harvested, during which time local school children receive a week off from school. The rice harvest coincides with China's second largest festival, the Mid-Autumn Festival. In winter, the farmers grow sweet potatoes, and there are several orange groves in the area.

Many farmers raised ducks to assist with fertilization, shared farm animals with other families, and took turns tending a single water buffalo. We saw a man walking a small horse covered with large sacks of rice and an elderly woman herding ducks by whacking them on the bum with a bamboo stick.

We watched a little girl, not more than two, attempt to sneak up on a large white cat (while her grandfather snoozed on a rickety bench under a tree). She tottered excitedly toward the cat, whereupon it casually stretched and sauntered a few feet away, seeming to know it could take its time. The adorable girl shrieked with delight, waved her chubby arms in the air, and hurried after the cat as fast as her short legs would carry her. Without realizing it, my eyes began to water, possibly more from amusement than pain.

Claire informed us that since 2006, Chinese farmers have not been required to pay taxes and have received a government subsidy for growing rice. While a challenging and highly physical lifestyle, the rice farming minority villagers appeared to be at ease and content living within their small, rural, tight-knit communities—and in many ways I envied and admired them.

Our prime view of the best terraced rice fields required a long, arduous hike, up endless and steep cobblestone steps, past several small minority villages. The farther we trekked the fewer tour groups and slowpokes there were. Eventually, it was just Claire, Chris, me, the locals, and a few stray dogs, one of which befriended us and followed us on the entire journey. The golden-brown dog with a white face and pointed ears looked exactly like a wild, Australian dingo. We named him Wang Chung after the eighties British pop band. Apparently, Wang Chung, means yellow bell, and is the first note in the Chinese classical musical scale. Who knew?

Throughout my four-year battle with infertility, in addition to Chris (who is the rational calm to my crazy emotional) my dogs were my constant companions. They never tired of my crying nor judged my emotional outbursts. They were always up for a walk to relieve stress, and they gave me something to nurture and love (and smother).

The day my dog, Jane, went to doggie heaven, was one of the worst days of my life and still haunts me. After her cancer diagnosis, we canceled a trip to Santa Fe to be with my family, then had to put her down on Thanksgiving Day (forever ruining the holiday for me). I insisted on staying in the room with her during the injection, not wanting her to be scared and alone with strangers when she died. I wrapped my arms around her frail, boney body but had to turn my face and look away. As soon as the emergency vet pushed the syringe I screamed, "I changed my mind, bring her back." I became hysterical and Chris had to carry me, kicking and screaming, out of the twenty-four-hour emergency vet.

To memorialize my beloved canine friend, I created a shrine to her in our bedroom. On a large picture ledge I placed her ashes, dog collar, and favorite toy (Red Squirrel), as well as, my favorite photo of us and a statue of St. Francis de Assisi (the patron saint of animals). After Jane's death, our other dog, Otis, and I weren't the same, but at least we still had each other and the happy memories of her climbing trees after squirrels (yes, Jane literally climbed trees, at least those with low branches or a slight lean).

Before leaving the Lóngsheng area, we stopped in a village for lunch and were given enough food to feed an army. We were served a delicious meal of sticky rice baked in a hollow piece of bamboo, mushroom soup, eggs with tomato, chicken with bamboo shoots, and beef with carrots and celery on a giant lazy Susan decorated with a picture of a dragon and a phoenix. Not wanting to be wasteful in a rural farm village, we stuffed ourselves until we were sick, only to be told afterward that all the leftovers were served to the farm animals.

In China's past, when food was scarce, a person's well-being was directly tied to the hunger level of his or her stomach. Therefore, Chinese people traditionally greeted each other with the phrase "*chi fan le ma?*" or "did you eat?" Today, the greeting is extended in kindness only; therefore, the polite response, even if you're hungry enough to eat a horse or snack on a dog, is always "Yes."

Throughout most of our meals in China, we were treated like royalty or guests at a wedding banquet, instantly served with a wide variety of anywhere from five to twenty-five small dishes. Other than the few times we dined alone, when feeling brave, bold and curious, we never had to navigate through a dangerously indecipherable menu. During tours our guides would occasionally order the regional specialty or share their favorite dish, but for the most part, we were presented with small dishes of everything the restaurant had to offer. Each meal was a feast of exotic options; we soon considered eating to be a big part of our experience.

According to Claire, "Sour food is from the East, sweet food is from the South, salty food is from the North, and spicy food is from the West." Chris and I agreed the cuisine of the North was more flavorful than the sweeter cuisine of the South, though we happily sampled everything and a lot of it—and we were quickly becoming fat and happy.

In most restaurants throughout China, tea was served first, regardless of whether it had been ordered. Drinking tea before a meal was thought to ease digestion. Tea was served before and after a meal but never during. If the teapot ran out, a slightly askew lid signaled the waitstaff more tea was needed. Cold dishes of beans, boiled eggs, shrimp, tofu or salads were usually served before the main meal, while rice was served together with the entrees. Soup was normally served after the main meal; then fruits and desserts were served before a final round of tea. Sadly they never served coffee. In Lóngsheng we got our first taste of wheat tea, which tasted just like it sounds. Wheat tea was like drinking a hot piece of toast.

One charming custom we noticed while dining in China was that instead of finding napkins stuffed into a metal dispenser or wrapped around bundles of silverware, we were given small, decorative packets of tissues. The tissue packets looked like bi-fold wallets with roughly five tissues neatly stacked under the flap on either side. Not only did these tissue packets make unique souvenirs, they helped me to survive my springtime allergies and got us out of numerous bathroom dilemmas where there was no toilet paper.

Over lunch one day, Claire told us that Chinese parents often predict the fortunes of their children based on how they hold their chopsticks. Those who hold their chopsticks close to the bottom will marry someone close to home; those who grip their chopsticks far from the base will marry and move away from home. She gave a tour to a German couple who both held their chopsticks very close to the bottom. It turned out they were neighbors before getting married. I could already picture myself gently encouraging my future daughter to hold her chopsticks close to the bottom.

We learned that when dining at a Chinese restaurant, always rest your chopsticks on the edge of your plate or on a chopstick rest, never on the table, which is considered unsanitary. Using your chopsticks as a pointing device or impromptu drumsticks is considered very rude and only children are allowed to use chopsticks to spear their food. If you become too full to finish your bowl of rice, never stand your chopsticks upright in the bowl, since the Chinese believe it resembles the sight of incense at a graveyard!

Perhaps one of the most cherished memories of our time spent in Guilin was our nightly walks.

One evening we walked all the way to Zhongshan Road, which was packed with giant shopping malls, fast food restaurants, and large department stores. The word *bustling* did not adequately describe the scene. It was more like "overwhelmingly intense, verging on sheer pandemonium" . . . and it was a Tuesday. While the sidewalks in Beijing were filled with mostly bicycles, the sidewalks in the downtown shopping area of Guilin were jam-packed with mopeds. They were blocking doorways, encroaching on commercial spaces, and impeding pedestrian foot traffic.

We were surprised to see upwards of four teenagers piled onto a single moped but were even more impressed by the badass little old lady traveling at breakneck speed on a pink moped down the center median. Entire families appeared to get around using a single moped at the same time, and mom and dad appeared to have no qualms with junior driving. Coming from a country where kids remain in booster seats until partway through grade school, we were shocked to see toddlers (not to mention dogs and chickens) riding around in milk crates attached to the fronts and rears of mopeds and motorcycles. However, Chris remembers riding around in the back of a van inside a playpen and driving from Maryland to Texas in the bed of the family pick-up truck with his sister in the 1970s. Plus, I have distinct memories of one of the mothers in my kindergarten car pool group steering with her knees while applying makeup, so who are we to judge?

Our favorite evening walks took us straight to the water. I can think of few things that are more romantic than an evening stroll around a lake with someone you love. Therefore, while staying in Guilin, Chris and I got into the delightful habit of taking a leisurely evening stroll around Rong Lake, which was truly the perfect end to each day.

One evening it had grown dark by the time we were walking back to the hotel, and it seemed like every single tree along the banks of Rong and Shan lake were filled with tiny, twinkling, fairy lights. The shores of the lakes glowed silver, gold, and green. The grand highlight to this nighttime light show was the twin Sun and Moon Buddhist Pagodas in the middle of Shan Lake. The nine-story Sun Pagoda is made of solid bronze, while the seven-story Moon Pagoda is made of wood and glazed tiles. At night, the Sun Pagoda glowed gold, while the Moon Pagoda sparkled silver.

Walking to the dock we watched boats cruise past the lit-up trees, glowing twin pagodas, and dancing fountains. Then we walked back to our hotel, hand in hand, in the glow of the ethereal lights, occasionally stopping for a romantic photo op and spur of the moment kiss.

Before our restorative trip to China, our happy newlywed days felt so far in the past; they seemed out of reach. We had completely forgotten our love for each other and what it meant to be a couple in our single-minded obsession with starting a family. Thanks to romantic, nightly walks and the mystical charm of Guilin's surreal landscapes, our hearts were beginning to reemerge from the shadows.

6

SNAKE WINE, ANYONE?

The hills and caves of Guilin are legendary, and we were fortunate enough to visit two of them, starting with Fubo Shan (Hill), which offered incredible views of the city of Guilin. The hill stands alone, half on land and half stretching out into the water. The portion stretching into the west bank of the Li River is part rocky cliff and partly covered with tall trees and thick foliage. Waves break against the hill and run back to the river; because of this the hill is often referred to as Wave-Subduing Hill.

During the Han dynasty, Ma Yuan, a royal official known as General Fubo, passed through Guilin while traveling south. According to a rather vague and fanciful legend, he was transporting herbs but was accused of secretly stashing pearls. To avoid conflict, he dumped all of his goods into the river, so Fubo Hill was named in his memory. Claire told us a more realistic story of beloved General Fubo. He greatly helped the people of Guilin by digging several canals.

At the base of the hill, there is a large cave called Huangzhu Dong or Pearl-Returning Cave, which used to only be accessible by boat. The story behind the cave's name is based on a tale of a fisherman who discovered an old man sleeping in the cave with a giant pearl by his side. The fisherman stole the pearl but then learned it belonged to the Dragon King, so he returned it, rather than face the king's wrath and his "devil waves."

If nothing else, these cryptic legends tell of the importance and value of pearls to the Chinese. More than anything, the Chinese have a fondness for round, white pearls due to their resemblance to the moon. One age-old Chinese myth claims pearls dropped from the sky after dragons fought amongst the clouds. In another ancient tale, a boy found a magic pearl, placed it in a jar with a bit of rice, and in the morning the jar was full of rice. When the villagers heard of the wonderous pearl, they tried to steal it. The boy swallowed the pearl to protect it and turned into a dragon. To this day, Chinese works of art often depict dragons guarding pearls.

Personally, I have a soft spot for pearls since they are associated with fertility and remind me of my prim and proper southern Grandmother Martha and her sister, my Great Aunt Doris. Doris gave me a string of pearls for my sixteenth birthday (which I didn't wear until my forties), and it's said Martha did her gardening in pearls and heels. As I struggled to become a mother, I started wearing my pearls as a symbolic connection to my ancestors and big, round bellies. Sadly, my great aunt died while we were trying to conceive, but thanks to a small inheritance from her, we were able to partially afford fertility treatments and adoption.

I simply couldn't imagine a life without children, since children had almost always been a part of my life. As a teen, I babysat all the neighborhood kids and worked at a trilingual summer camp. I paid my expenses during college teaching preschool; then after graduation I worked as an au pair for a French family in Paris. I've volunteered to work with abused kids in the social services system and taught privileged kids on vacation to ski. In addition to working as a journalist, I received a master's in elementary education, taught early childhood literacy and specialized in dyslexia. I have dedicated the better part of my life to working with other people's children.

The possibility of never having my own children was beyond devastating. I literally thought my life had no value without motherhood and I had no purpose without children. I often felt completely lost, with no direction, drifting through life, as I waited for a child.

Inside the Pearl-Returning Cave, a stalactite rock formation named Sword-Testing Rock hung from the ceiling. The rock was wider at the top and grew narrower toward the bottom, like a melting icicle dripping down toward the ground. From afar the pillar appeared to touch the ground, but upon closer inspection, the stalactite stopped roughly one inch before reaching the ground—as if the tip of the rock were sliced off. According to legend, General Fubo tested the might of his sword by cutting the stone pillar, which left a small crevice at its base. Visitors were supposed to rub the bottom of the stalactite for good luck. The base of the rock was completely smooth from centuries of being rubbed.

Further into the Pearl-Returning cavern is Thousand-Buddha Cave, were there are more than two hundred Buddhist statues and more than one hundred carved inscriptions. It was thought to be good luck to stick your hand through a hole in a rock, reaching out past a guardrail, to rub the knee of a large statue of Buddha carved into the cliff wall, facing the river. I rubbed his knee till it shone and wished with all my might for a child.

When traveling, you can be almost whoever you want to be, break from your norm and try out another persona. In China, I became a blonde, American celebrity (at least the locals seemed to think so).

Throughout our time in China, my long, golden hair drew a lot of attention. While we encountered lots of other Asian tourists, we saw very few Caucasians, even fewer Americans and hardly any blondes. According to Claire, millions of Chinese travel during springtime, plus lots of Korean and Japanese people flock to China year-round to play golf. Since both Korea and Japan are small countries, land is precious and therefore golf courses are rare and expensive. Whereas expansive China offers Asian tourists a wide variety of golf courses at a lower cost.

In Guilin, a group of young Korean women wearing pastel plaid golf outfits complete with giant pom-pom hats asked to take a photo with me. They placed me in the center and gathered around me on all sides. At a mere five feet eight inches, I still towered over them. They giggled uncontrollably, all made the peace sign, and took roughly thirty photographs.

Each day of our trip, I was asked to join in photos. I was asked to hold, and even kiss, babies. Other times I noticed some random person taking a picture of me. Several times I felt the shadow of curious onlookers peeking over my shoulder to see the strange letters I was writing in my journal. While I was greatly amused and flattered by all the attention, I was surprised by the level of forwardness of the Chinese and other Asian tourists. They had no qualms whatsoever touching my hair, following me, and simply staring at me for uncomfortably long periods of time, like I was an exotic creature that escaped from the zoo.

In my youth, during a Eurail trip throughout Europe, I sat next to a young Japanese girl on a train who was obsessed with not just my bright blue eyes, but my eyelids! She informed me that Asians don't have a fold in their eyelids and that many Asian women were going through plastic surgery to get a "Western fold." The female desire to be taller, thinner, and possess bigger boobs seems universal, but this was a new one. Personally, I've always craved darker eyebrows, eyelashes, and skin tone. (The downside to being a natural blonde, in my opinion, is the fairness and freckles that come with it.) But thanks to this eye-opening experience, I now have an appreciation for my Western eyelid folds.

After hiding in the dark for years, feeling ashamed and faulty due to infertility, it felt wonderful to be admired. While traveling in China, I felt more attractive, younger, and vibrant, but most of all intriguing and desirable. It was a truly confidence boosting, cathartic rush to shine in the spotlight (if only temporarily).

Guilin's most famous landmark, Xiang Bi Shan or Elephant Trunk Hill, was one of my best-beloved spots. Located at the confluence of the Li and Taohua (Peach Blossom) Rivers, the hill looks like a giant elephant drinking water from the river. The elephant's trunk, legs, and lower torso are rock, while its back is made of the lush foliage on top of the hill. It is featured on all travel brochures, restaurant menus, and countless souvenirs.

The naturally formed arch between the elephant's trunk and front legs made the Water Moon Cave. The cave was unique in that it arched over a river and a stream trickled through the center of the cave. Plus, the cave walls were carved with more than fifty inscriptions, the earliest dating from the Song dynasty

(960-1279). At night, the cave and its reflection together created a bright moon image on the water.

It is said that Elephant Trunk Hill is the embodiment of Puxian, the Buddha of Wisdom. Long ago Puxian served the emperor but suffered wounds during a battle and was stranded in Guilin. A local couple saved his life, and during his recovery, he fell in love with Guilin. He decided to remain in the city. Rather than return to the royal palace, he turned into Elephant Trunk Hill, thereby becoming a lasting symbol of his beloved Guilin.

The emperor bestowed the people of Guilin with a pagoda, known as the Puxian Pagoda, to protect them from evil. The brick tower, which sits on top of Elephant Trunk Hill, is a place to worship Samantabhadra, a beloved bodhisattvas, often seen riding atop an elephant.

Elephants have always been one of my favorite animals. They are capable of serious damage yet choose to remain gentle giants. They are intelligent and emotional, strict vegetarians, and friends to all other animals and humans. In Chinese, the word for elephant (*xiàng*) has a similar pronunciation to the word for lucky (*xìngyùn*) and therefore elephants are thought to be very auspicious.

Love Island sits in the middle of the Li River, just north of Elephant Trunk Hill. The island got its name due to the numerous love-themed statues that decorate it, including a statue of a kissing couple (the man wears a pointed straw hat), a mother and child (entwined together in a single piece of stone), and two hands interwoven in friendship. Claire insisted on taking cheesy photos of Chris and I standing next to (and mimicking) each love themed statue on Love Island.

We randomly happened upon a group of Zhuang minority students who were dressed in colorful, embroidered costumes and practicing native dances, which they performed during the harvest and New Year's festivals. They held hands in circles, with an inner and outer circle of dancers spinning around. The Chinese teens looked radiantly happy and their dance appeared to be an expression of pure joy, all of which made me smile. I even joined in the fun with an impromptu dance lesson.

In addition to whimsical statues and dancing teenagers, Love Island featured numerous ginkgo trees and osmanthus flowers, the official tree and flower of Guilin. Ginkgo trees are often called grandpa and grandson trees. Legend tells of a grandfather who planted a ginkgo tree that did not grow until the day his grandson was born. The wide leaves look like Chinese fans. Claire told us that she used ginkgo leaves as bookmarks during grade school. Ginkgo is thought to be good for blood pressure and a healthy heart and is a hot seller in traditional herbal pharmacies throughout China. The osmanthus flower is a popular Guilin souvenir item, sold as osmanthus tea, jelly, cake, essential oil, and fragrant sachets.

The Chinese draw direct connections between floral and human nature and believe that flowers never lie. Plums are a symbol of longevity and happy marriage, cherry blossoms impart happiness, pomegranates bring abundant prosperity (namely many children), and lotus flowers symbolize pureness of heart. Happily married couples are often described as two lotus flowers on one stem. Even China's major religions have a floral pairing: Confucianism is paired with pine, Buddhism with bamboo or lotus, and Taoism with plum or peaches.

In China, peaches are a symbol for love. It is said that if you want to find love, take a bath at night along the banks of the Peach Blossom River and your dream will come true. Having already found the love of my life, I wondered if this legend could be applied toward having a baby and considered running naked, in the rain, along the banks of the Taohua River one evening. When in China.

Since haggling in China is a competitive sport, at which we failed miserably, we quickly gave up shopping at street markets and mega stores and resorted to almost nightly visits to Chinese convenience stores. We found the Chinese version of a 7-Eleven to be a welcome relief from the magnitude of department stores and the chaos of street markets in China. The convenience store clerks never bothered us nor harassed us to buy anything. We were free to wander the store and explore the racks of exotic Chinese necessities and oddities in peace.

After each convenience store visit, we added to our growing collection of kitschy Chinese knickknacks: a travel mah-jongg set, a Chairman Mao car air freshener, a Chinese opera mask bottle opener, and a large collection of Chinese talismans and charms (two cranes for a happy union, ancient coins with a hole in the center, and an absolutely fake jade pendant with the Chinese character for mother).

Each night, we would agree on the most intriguing desserts to share, usually a Little Debbie or Hostess style Chinese snack cake. We considered nightly desserts to be an important cultural experience (at least that's what we told ourselves as we packed on the pounds). We also acquired a wide variety of exotic and colorful Chinese candy (again, for research purposes). Our frequent liquor purchases began as a cultural science experiment but grew into a serious souvenir bottle collection.

It quickly became clear that no matter what type of alcohol we chose, solely based on the appeal of its bottle and label design, it all tasted like a fiery combination of battery acid, Drano, and windshield washer fluid (not that I've actually tasted any of these liquids). Against our natural instincts, we tossed a lot of alcohol down the hotel sink drain. The varieties of *huangjiu* (yellow rice wine) and sorghum based *baiju* (Chinese vodka) were cheap, made for a fun night, and the empty bottles provided us with one of our most memorable souvenir collections.

We examined liquor bottles with pieces of ginseng and other roots and herbs floating around like alcoholic snow globes. We saw bottles with pickled bees, scorpions, centipedes, and snakes. That's right, one bottle had a whole venomous snake coiled up on the bottom and another featured a snake zigzagging up to the top. The Chinese seemed convinced that poisonous animals protect babies, cure blood circulation illnesses, and improve men's virility and stamina. In addition to snake, eel, and baby mouse wine, there was even a three-penis liquor, allegedly made from seal, deer, and dog penises. (It would take an awful lot to convince me to partake of this "cock" tail.)

We started our souvenir bottle collection in Beijing with a squat, oval-shaped, beige bottle decorated with an opera mask on each side. Then in Xi'an, we acquired an earthy, terra-cotta vase etched with Chinese characters, sealed with red wax, and topped with a square of leather. In Guilin, we purchased our favorite bottle of alcohol. Our selection had nothing to do with its taste, which was like lighter fluid. Instead, we were thrilled that the small, pottery vessel was in the exact shape of Elephant Trunk Hill.

We had no idea what any of the Chinese characters on the bottles meant, nor what type of toxic fluid they held within, so we simply chose the most exotic, inexpensive, or sometimes beautiful bottle. Then we would hurry back to our hotel room giggling like teenage kids, who just snuck booze out of their parent's seriously bizarre liquor cabinet.

During one impromptu late-night outing to the convenience store, we searched for a birthday cake to appease our guilt from learning that Claire had spent her entire birthday with us. We presented her with three different mini cakes, as well as gifts from home that we brought for each tour guide, including an English language crossword puzzle book, a Rocky Mountain refrigerator magnet, a bag of chocolate bear poop, a Denver Broncos keychain, and a holiday ornament of a moose riding a sled.

At first, Claire refused to accept our gifts, and we assumed she felt awkward taking gifts from clients. However, we later discovered that it is customary for the Chinese to refuse a gift at least once, if not several times, to show humility. While they likely appreciate and desire the gift, according to their culture, they must first say no to be polite. A similar stance is taken in regard to compliments, since immediately accepting a compliment is seen as a sign of vanity.

Claire explained that she didn't celebrate the day of her birth because in China everyone shares a communal birthday and birthday parties are reserved for children and seniors.

We learned that in China, birthdays are generally celebrated at one month, one year, sometimes six years, and then every decade starting with fifty. Turning sixty in China is a huge milestone, since it is the completion of the full cycle of the twelve Chinese zodiac astrological signs and a brand-new life starts at sixty-one. For all other years, mass birthdays are traditionally celebrated on the seventh day of the Chinese New Year. This day is considered everybody's birthday, and everyone automatically advances one year.

At birth, a Chinese infant is already considered to be one year old, based on time spent in the womb. Therefore, a child born on New Year's Eve could be considered two years old, just eight days later. In the past, a child wasn't considered a person until the age of three. Instead he or she was only a continuation of their parents, and if the child died before three, it wasn't given a funeral. Granted infant mortality rates were much higher centuries ago, I still had a hard time with this concept since I had grieved the loss and memorialized a child that wasn't even born.

To honor a child's first one hundred days and officially announce their birth, Chinese parents throw a big party where they serve hard-boiled eggs that are dyed red for happiness and luck and pickled gingerroot to represent strong family roots.

To celebrate a child's first birthday, a traditional game called *zhuā zhōu*, or drawing lots, believed to have originated during the Three Kingdoms period, was played to determine a child's future. The child was presented with several items including a book, a flute, coins, jewelry, flowers, and other objects supplied by the guests. Then the parents, relatives and guests would anxiously await the child's highly symbolic choice, as the chosen item was believed to indicate the child's future.

For example, the selection of an abacus meant the child would be successful in business, while a bowl of rice indicated the child would become a farmer (or maybe the poor kid was just hungry). The most highly regarded option was a book that predicted a future scholar and meant pride and fame for the whole family. I would be very surprised if any baby chose a dusty old book over a shiny metal coin or a colorful, sweet-smelling flower.

My father used to say, "One of the greatest blessings in life is to enjoy your work, since it ceases to be work when you like what you do, are good at it, and make a living you can be proud of." Wise words, except for the fact that my father was a stressed-out workaholic. He steered my future throughout my youth and pushed me toward international business during college. I was well into my twenties before I was brave enough to tell him I wanted to be a journalist (and when I did, he said, "good luck making a living"). I can only imagine how he would have reacted to my one-year-old self-choosing a pencil—for shame, the horror, say it isn't so!

I simply hoped my future daughter would follow her dreams toward whatever career she was destined for and that by following her natural instincts and talents it would bring her success and happiness.

7

UNDER THE BANYAN TREE

We boarded a flat-bottom, two-story boat in the early morning hours during a light rain. A lovely mist blanketed the river and the surrounding mountains.

Chris and I were about to take a scenic, four-hour cruise along the Li River from Guilin to Yangshuo. The Chinese have a saying about the Li River: "One hundred kilometers of Li River, one hundred kilometers of art gallery."

We couldn't agree more. Without question, the Li River cruise was our absolute favorite activity and fondest memory of China. The slow and steady river cruise past endless natural beauty was pure heaven (even for someone with severe motion sickness).

There simply aren't enough words to describe the haunting beauty of Southern China's Yangshuo County. The eighty-seven photos we took of the emerald mountains rising above the shimmering river, all shrouded in mist, don't do the intoxicating allure of the Li River Valley justice. It was magical, surreal—the stuff fairytales are made of. If dragons exist, they surely live amongst the green hills, crystal waters, and mysterious caves of Yangshuo County.

Along the banks of the Li Jiang were odd shaped crags, deep pools, rushing springs, large caves, towering peaks, variegated cliffs, plunging waterfalls, and incredible landscapes filled with bamboo forests, duck farms, and fields of rice. Many of the lush green hills and white karst rock formations had fascinating names like Writing Brush Peak, River Snail Hill, and Celestial Being Hill.

Yearning for a Husband Rock was said to look like a mother with a child on her back, looking out across the water for her husband who has gone to the city to help build the Great Wall. The huge Crown Cave was said to resemble an ancient Chinese imperial crown when in autumn the surrounding foliage turns to purple and gold. The cave looked very deep and we could just barely make out small rafts floating inside and little children playing at the edge of darkness. Next, we saw the Painted Hill of Nine Horses, where some people claim to see the images of nine horses in the limestone rock. I only saw three horses, but my attention was elsewhere, as I was determined to spot a dragon.

Han Yu, a poet from the Tang dynasty, painted the perfect image of the Li River with his words, "The river winds like a blue silk ribbon, while the hills erect like green jade hairpins."

At one point, I became intrigued by one of our neighbors on the river: a teenaged boy who stood atop what can barely be described as a raft, consisting of only five bamboo poles tied together and being only about two feet wide. He pulled up alongside the tour boat and attempted to sell fruit. Several passengers leaned precariously over the edge of the boat to purchase oranges.

I pondered how the raft, which sat only an inch or two above the waterline, managed not to submerge in the wake of our boat. We watched an old fisherman rowing upriver on a similar raft and saw that more than half of the vessel, including the fisherman's feet, was submerged under water. Only the front and back tips of the raft, where the bamboo poles curved upwards, and a large crate in the center, were visible above the water.

When it comes to water vessels in China—anything goes. Of the hundreds of rafts, we observed on the Li River, some rafts had curved tips at the front and rear, while others only curved in back; but the majority were completely flat. We even saw a few bamboo rafts with small motors. On closer inspection, I determined that the hollow bamboo poles were plugged (but the crafts still seemed to defy the physical law of buoyancy, and I questioned whether even Archimedes would have been mystified). I wondered how the straw baskets perched on top of the flat rafts didn't float away as none of them appeared to be tied down. Perhaps, I thought, they filled the baskets with rocks, when empty of goods. It helped that the waters of the Li River were perfectly calm and as slow as molasses in January, as my daddy used to say. I wondered if the Chinese had a word for "white-water rapids," or "gentle waves" for that matter.

As we continued our enchanting journey along the Li River, we passed by a floating fish market underneath several pop-up tents where locals selected fish directly from tubs on the backs of rafts anchored along the shore. Numerous large, blackish-grey cormorant birds rested upon the rafts, as their fisherman owners made the rounds and no doubt haggled for a higher price.

Since roughly 960 AD, cormorant fishing has been a traditional fishing method in China. Fishermen use trained cormorant birds to fish in the shallow water of the Li River. To control the birds, fishermen tie a snare near the base of their throat, preventing them from swallowing any large fish. Once the cormorant has caught a fish, the fisherman pulls it back to the boat on a cord; the bird spits up the fish and then receives a small reward.

According to Claire, most Chinese fisherman have a great respect for their cormorant birds and treat them as beloved pets. We saw dozens of cormorants on cords sitting atop flat bamboo rafts and small boats with impossibly low berths, some just tall enough for tiny windows.

Cormorant fishing was once a successful industry but is now primarily used to entertain tourists. A perfect example of this was Old Father China, a local fisherman turned entrepreneur, who greeted tourist boats at the Yangshuo dock. He wore a pointed straw hat and black cotton jumpsuit, and across the top of his shoulders he carried a bamboo pole with a large cormorant bird perched on each end. Apparently, he made a small fortune charging tourists for a photo of him and his pets. I should know, I paid him ten yuan, which was roughly $1.50, for one photo, albeit a very charming and memorable one.

One of the best aspects of traveling is meeting new people, learning their stories, and sharing travel adventures together. I'll never forget meeting a man in an elevator in Beijing who lived in Australia but is from New Mexico, then seeing him and his wife again while shopping in the Muslin Quarter of Xi'an. Sometimes it's a very small and delightful world!

During our cruise on the Li River, we shared a long table with several other tourists for a greasy buffet lunch (which surely would have resulted in nausea regardless of being served on a boat). Our tablemates consisted of a German couple, an Italian twosome, and a couple from China. The Germans, a doctor and a nurse from Hamburg, just so happened to stay at our hotel and joined us for breakfast the following day for more cross-cultural bonding.

At the table behind us, a group of Eastern European looking women, all wrapped in scarves and shawls, sang folk songs. The somber and sad sounding melodies, which to my ears sounded a bit like the American negro spiritual "Swing Low Sweet Chariot" in Yiddish, seemed more appropriate for a boat crossing to Ellis Island than a scenic cruise down the Li River. Then again, "Swing Low Sweet Chariot" has become the unofficial anthem of the England National Rugby Team.

Throughout our travels in China, we came across tourists from all over the world, including England, Switzerland, Australia, Sweden, Spain, Korea, Japan, and Iceland. While the vast majority of tourists were Chinese and other Asians, the second largest group of tourists wandering around China seemed to be French (based on my formerly fluent but fading French).

One of my greatest regrets is not studying Spanish during my school years. Growing up in New Mexico, I was surrounded by Spanish speakers and didn't find Spanish to be interesting. So I chose to learn French; to me, it was more exotic and romantic (and I wasn't thinking in terms of my future career or lifestyle). I worked for years to master the French language, used it briefly during my year spent in Paris as a nanny, only to completely lose all my hard-earned skills because I no longer use or practice the language. Meanwhile, I am frustrated daily by the fact that I can't speak Spanish with my friends, neighbors, and community (not to mention my entire family, which ali speak fluent Spanish). Once again, I'm the misfit not quite fitting in as a former French speaker in a community and family of Spanish speakers. Now as an adult, I am struggling to learn Spanish, but it is much more difficult, and I speak a disgraceful, French/Spanish mélange.

In terms of Chinese, I've managed to retain a few phrases and several random words in Mandarin. I hope to learn more Mandarin, but my aging brain already can barely remember French and is struggling to learn Spanish, so I'm fighting a losing battle.

None the less, according to my husband, I can strike up a conversation with anyone, anytime, anywhere, and in any language. I've mixed ancient private school Latin, rusty French and rudimentary Spanish in an effort to converse with Italians. On more than one occasion, I've had a lengthy discussion with a stranger via sketch pad doodles and elaborate pantomime. During our engagement trip to Greece, Chris stepped on a sea urchin, and the lifeguard used hand gestures to indicate that Chris should take his dick out and pee on his foot. It was like a scene from *Friends* and was definitely a conversation across language barriers that raised a few eyebrows.

As someone who enjoys meeting unexpected and interesting people, I've started conversations with random strangers on buses, trains, and planes; while waiting in a queue; and during visits to the ladies' room. While visiting Spain, I toured Seville with two German guys I met on a bus and explored Madrid with a Japanese girl I sat next to on a train. I celebrated my birthday in Granada with some Dutch exchange students I met at a couscous restaurant. I explored Barcelona with a blue-eyed blonde girl from Chile I met at a youth hostel (who became outraged when locals assumed she was also American and spoke English to her).

Throughout my life and travels, I have butchered multiple languages, offended a wide variety of foreigners, and made a complete ass of myself due to my desperate need to communicate. (I'm seriously that outgoing and curious.) I could have a stimulating conversation with a brick wall, obtain vital information from a house plant, and make friends with the dead.

✿

As we glided past the many picturesque villages along the banks of the Li River, I began to wonder if our future child would be from a rural fishing or farming village, a massive modern city, or the magnificent mountains or deserts of China.

We floated past the tiny village of Yangdi, named after the hill that rises above the town and looks like an upside-down goat's hoof. We also saw the town of Caoping, a Muslim village with mainly Hui minority people. Several small children splashed and played along the shore in their underwear. A group of women with babies on their backs and wicker baskets on their heads gathered along the water's edge to wash clothes in the river.

Perhaps, our future daughter would be from one of these charming rural towns along the banks of the Li River. Or she might be a child of the vast Gobi Desert or born amongst a backdrop of breathtaking mountains in Tibet. Maybe she would come from the misty forests of central China where pandas roam or be born into the chaotic energy of one of China's cosmopolitan cities. Would she have the big forehead and small eyes of the Mongolian people of the North or the dark skin and short stature common amongst the citizens of Southern China? Would she be a part of the Han majority or from one of China's small minority groups, however unlikely. Would she be from a family of practicing Buddhists, Christians, or Muslims?

How remotely similar or vastly different would the place and circumstances of her birth be from her upbringing in the United States? Would we be given any details about our adopted daughter's heritage, and would we be able to faithfully impart aspects of her Chinese ancestry? As much as the history and culture of China fascinated me, I was overwhelmed and intimidated by the responsibility and challenges of raising an orphan from a foreign country—but also alive with excitement and wonder.

I've often marveled at how mature, highly educated, mentally stable, and financially prepared infertile couples must jump through hoops, invest a fortune, and wait half a lifetime for a baby. Meanwhile teens around the world are getting pregnant in the backs of cars, on their first time, to their dismay. It's almost comical, if it weren't so damned infuriating.

When we shared our plan to adopt from China, some people criticized us and asked why we weren't adopting from the United States. While we considered a domestic adoption, we had heard too many heartbreaking stories of domestic adoptions that fell through at the last minute. Being older and having already suffered through more than two years of failed fertility treatments and miscarriages, we were highly emotional and anxious and simply couldn't take the risk. At the time, due to China's stringent population control measures, thousands of baby girls were being given up for adoption, and we had hoped for a better guarantee of a healthy baby, in a timely manner, with fewer complications—but we were wrong.

Many of the success stories of happy families prominently featured throughout our adoption agency included blended families, with both adopted and conceived children. The walls of our adoption agency were filled with adorable family portraits featuring giant, fat American babies alongside tiny, delicate Asian orphans. We hoped to become one of those radiant family units with several kids, conceived and adopted, Caucasian and Asian (or any other race), boy or girl—none of it mattered to us as long as we got a family.

We had hoped to visit an orphanage somewhere along our travels through China. We figured as future parents of a Chinese orphan, officially on a waiting list with all the appropriate legal documentation, it would have been no big deal—but we were wrong. Our adoption agency informed us that the Chinese government absolutely forbid visits to orphanages and no amount of pleading phone calls and heartfelt letters made any difference. Not only were we deeply frustrated and disappointed, we were left to ponder why the Chinese orphanages were off limits.

The closed-door policy raised endless, frightening questions. We assumed the worst, that the conditions were deplorable, and our future daughter and other innocent children were suffering. We had visions of a Charles Dicken's–style orphanage and nightmares about the Spanish horror film *The Orphanage*, which I wished I could erase. We began to worry about the general lack of information. We had already waited two years for a baby and had no idea why it was taking so long and whether or not our future child was being well cared for.

The thought of our baby possibly suffering while waiting for a home, while we agonized waiting to provide a home was too much to bear. It was torture thinking our child might be so close and in need of our help and yet so far. While it was difficult to remain hopeful and keep blindly moving forward through our fears, the most we could do was learn everything we could about China's history and culture in preparation for becoming conscientious parents of a Chinese orphan—and continue to wait.

As our cruise drew to a close, we found the ancient boat dock and grand entrance to the city of Yangshuo absolutely breathtaking. A white stone, double staircase led to a large platform bustling with activity and filled with souvenir carts and snack stands (and photo ops with Old Father China). An arched doorway through a gate with a pavilion on top led directly to Foreigner Street, a.k.a. West Street, which ran from the river straight through the heart of town. A waterfall, eager to meet the Li River, rushed over large boulders to one side of the grand entrance. Pavilions and tiny temples hid amongst the thick foliage on the surrounding hills, the largest of which, Longtou Hill, set the backdrop for the charming town.

As we got off the boat, Claire announced, "Welcome to Yangshuo, the joy of Guangxi Providence, China's most beautiful, rural fishing village." We couldn't wait to breathe some fresh air, gain some personal space, and relax in the peaceful, quiet countryside.

However, as we looked around, it quickly became clear that while Yangshuo was lovely, it was no longer a village. Maybe a hundred years ago you could have called it a village, but these days, Yangshuo was a bustling tourist destination and mecca for rock climbers.

We asked Claire the population of Yangshuo, and she nonchalantly answered, "three hundred thousand," which is fourteen times the size of our hometown in Colorado.

Yangshuo proved once again that in China, even rural, off-the-beaten-path, former fishing villages are huge compared to most of the world's standards. That being said, for a large town in China, Yangshuo was relatively quiet, clean, and developed (by Chinese standards).

Yangshuo was well known amongst travelers in Southern China. Due to the relatively high number of foreign visitors, many locals spoke some English, and most street signs were in both Chinese and English. Plus, the stunning natural beauty and laid-back scene in Yangshuo had attracted lots of ex-patriots. In addition to the fabulous Li River cruise and gorgeous bike tours of the countryside, the Yangshuo region offers world-class rock climbing. The most famous crag is Moon Hill, but climbers also flock to Twin Gates, Baby Frog, and Wine Bottle Cliff, to name a small few.

The town of Yangshuo even has celebrity status having been featured in the movie *Star Wars Episode III: Revenge of the Sith* as Chewbacca's home plant of Kashyyyk and as a level in the landmark 1993 video game *Doom*. So maybe our loudly snoring neighbor at our hotel in Xi'an really was Chewie en route to his familial home in Yangshuo?

As we meandered through an open market and shops on West Street, I was thrilled to find a lovely porcelain ox figurine with a lucky orange on its back, seated upon a red, silk cushion.

It just so happens that Chris and I were both born during the Year of the Ox, and we were traveling in China together, thirty-five years later, during the Year of the Ox. So it seemed fitting to purchase an homage to the mighty ox.

Those born under the Chinese zodiac sign of the ox are said to be unpretentious and uncompromising, as well as diligent and devoted. They work hard no matter the number and difficulty of obstacles, definitely the character traits needed to survive two years of fertility treatments and waiting two years and counting on an international adoption. Plus, as water ox, we're able to endure hardship—got that right.

I have always identified more with my Chinese zodiac sign than my Western sign of Scorpio, which has always struck me as rather dark and ominous. My Scorpio horoscopes seem solely concerned with power, money, and sex. Based on my Western sign, I am a conniving, backstabbing, bloodthirsting, power hungry, sex fiend. So as unglamorous as an ox may be, it's better than a deadly scorpion!

The ancient Chinese took animal zodiac signs very seriously, sometimes using them to decide matters of life and death. Detailed horoscopes have long been the key to successful arranged marriages. Many potential partnerships have ended in ruin upon discovery of signs in direct opposition, such as Monkey and Rooster, Pig and Dog, or Tiger and Rabbit.

A persistent Rat is likely to annoy an independent Horse, while a discreet Rabbit might be bothered by a candid Rooster and a demanding Dragon is sure to overwhelm a laid-back Dog. But whatever you do, don't put two Roosters under the same roof; according to the Chinese zodiac rules of compatibility, they're likely to peck each other to death.

According to the Chinese zodiac, Oxen match perfectly with Rats, Snakes, and Roosters but should avoid Tigers, Dragons, Horses, and Sheep. Oxen are said to be reserved and shy about courting but are serious about committed and balanced marriages.

Apparently, a marriage of two Oxen is predicted as average but compatible since they share the same goals and together strive for a good standard of living. After fifteen years of happy marriage, I respectfully beg to differ with the Ox marriage rating of average. I believe a fellow uncompromising Ox is the perfect companion on a long and difficult journey to parenthood—those less determined and stubborn than an Ox would surely have given up.

Yangshuo may mean "Bright New Moon," in Chinese, but both the moon and the sun chose to remain hidden during our entire visit. While the rain was a bit of an inconvenience, the accompanying mist resulted in mysterious, ethereal photos and a permeating sense of fantasy, wonder, and romance.

Upon our afternoon arrival in Yangshuo, we were supposed to take a leisurely bike ride to Moon Hill. Sadly, the spring weather chose not to cooperate, and we had to travel by car, which wasn't the exhilarating and liberating adventure I had hoped for.

However, Moon Hill was very impressive. The hill rises to a rounded point, has a rocky cliff face, and foliage along the top. Moon Hill is best known for the natural, karst, 164-foot arch that cuts through its center, hence the name. American rock climber, Todd Skinner, established the first climbing route on the arch in 1992, which he dubbed Moonwalker. The walk to the base of the arch was easy and quick, but there was a fee, and souvenir and snack vendors followed us the entire way—ruining all hopes for a nature-inspired epiphany.

While Moon Hill was for rock climbers, romantics flocked to the Big Banyan Tree to propose, celebrate an anniversary, or simply cuddle. As for those who were looking for love, the locals claimed a wish for love came true under the ancient tree. Ever since the tree was featured in the 1960s Chinese musical *Liu Sanjie*, in which Liu Sanjie shows her love for A'niu by giving him an embroidered ball under the tree, the tree has been associated with romance. The Zhuang minority considered the roughly fourteen-hundred-year-old banyan tree to be an immortal God Tree.

The banyan tree is roughly fifty-six feet tall and twenty-three feet wide and looks like a giant leafy umbrella, fully capable of blocking the sun's rays with its thick foliage. Or as we discovered, the perfect shelter from the rain and setting for our own romantic interlude under a Chinese God Tree. While on vacation, away from the hell of infertility treatments and long wait to adopt and surrounded by enchanting natural beauty, I suddenly became as amorous as a teenager with her first crush.

While visiting the Big Banyan Tree, I became secretly enamored with an elderly Chinese couple sitting on a park bench next to the ancient tree. They didn't appear to say a word to each other, but it seemed they didn't need to. They simple sat, side by side, holding hands and sharing the same umbrella.

I have many fond memories of visiting large, beautiful parks throughout China. My favorite one was Tiantan Park in Beijing. We went during the early morning hours to get a glimpse into the daily rituals of seniors, before hordes of tourists invaded at a more reasonable hour. Elderly men practiced calligraphy, writing Chinese characters on large paving stones with foam tipped brushes dipped in water. In covered courtyards, small groups of seniors played chess, dominos, and cards (chess being one of the favorite activities of Chinese seniors and often played in boisterous teams). Several locals practiced Tai Chi, which was simply mesmerizing and beautiful to observe. We watched couples waltzing and large groups of seniors in ornate costumes practicing traditional Chinese minority dances. Groups of more than one hundred elderly Chinese often sang folk songs together. Many locals played shuttlecock, flew kites, and twirled ribbons.

We often observed large crowds of elderly Chinese vigorously clapping their hands and were surprised to learn that clapping was considered a form of exercise in China, since it was believed to circulate blood.

Most of all, the contented elders of China sat and talked while drinking copious amounts of tea.

According to Claire, China is a great place to be elderly since seniors are very respected and cared for. Filial piety and respect for elders is a source of virtue amongst Chinese. There's even a saying in China, "If you do not obey your elders, you will live ten years less." In Chinese families, elders are held in the highest esteem. They are seated first, served first, eat first, depart first, and always get the final word.

I've always admired countries where ancestors are honored, the elderly are esteemed, and generations of family live together. I grew up mostly lacking the wisdom, guidance, and love of grandparents. My paternal grandfather died many years before I was born, while my paternal grandmother died when I was "knee-high to a junebug" (as my Great Aunt Doris used to say). A visit with my maternal grandparents required a two-day road trip, therefore I saw them every two years or so, and was one of fifteen grandkids. My closest relationship was with my Great Aunt Doris, who I spoke with regularly—on the phone.

One of my greatest fears is growing old. I'm terrified of losing my physical abilities and mental capacities (and it doesn't help that my father had Parkinson's disease). I desperately hope to grow old alongside my husband, with children (who want) to support and care for me and grandchildren to teach, pamper, and adore.

I was completely enthralled as I watched the seniors of China going about their typical morning routines in local parks, full of comradery, merriment, and ancient customs. This quiet observation of daily life in a foreign country is one of my most beloved memories of China. For in those peaceful moments, I left my world and its troubles behind and was fully transported to another place and time.

That evening, Chris and I turned the romance level up a few degrees with our first fancy dinner—on our own. Until then, our dinners had consisted of prepaid dinner shows, cheap and easy street food, and two meals on an airplane. It was a fun and challenging adventure selecting dishes for ourselves and after a few local beers proved to be a romantic date night.

We dined at the popular Meiyou Restaurant on West Street. A sign out front read "Meiyou Warm Beer, Meiyou Lousy Food, Meiyou Rip-offs, Meiyou Pay FEC, Meiyou Bad Service." Turns out, *Meiyou* in Chinese means "Don't Have."

Chris chose the local delicacy Beer Fish, beer battered black carp caught by a cormorant and served in an ornate wok with dragon feet filled with a bright red spicy broth and huge chunks of green bell pepper.

According to our waiter, who spoke heavily accented but near-perfect English, there are several important steps to preparing a proper beer fish. First, a fresh, live carp must be caught from the Li River, so that it had the contentment of living in a place with green hills and clear water. Second, the fish must be cooked in Yangshuo with water from the Li River. Last, and most important, the fish must be cut without scrapping its scales, fried in local camellia oil, and soaked with local beer.

He added that the dish was very spicy and many foreigners couldn't take the heat. Chris, who puts heartburn-inducing and deadly ass-blasting amounts of hot sauce on just about everything, didn't flinch and said it was his favorite meal (aside from the spicy fried green beans, of course). While he loved the local dish, he hardly made a dent in the full-size wok filled to the brim and was sad to let the leftovers go uneaten.

I had curry noodles and fried rice. The fried rice came wrapped inside a "bowl" made of scrambled eggs and when unwrapped the egg bowl looked like a yellow flower. A pile of tiny, cherry tomatoes sat in the middle of the rice to give the added effect of red seeds. We both enjoyed a few light lagers (Liquan, brewed in Guilin) and jasmine tea. The meal was delicious, generous, and cost only twenty-eight dollars, a pittance compared to any nice date night in the States.

As we sat, alongside a huge window in the second-floor restaurant getting drunk on local beer, we had great fun watching the people on West Street and creating fake dialogues.

"Dude, do you know where I can find the Grungy Backpacker Hostel?

"Yo, the face of Moon Hill was gnarly. I'm wrecked."

"Did you hear there's some ol' tree that gets people horny?"

"Check out this bitchin photo I took of some old fisherman and his pet birds."

"Hey, man, want some herb?"

By the time our dessert of sweet sesame seed balls arrived, and I finished my second beer (while Chris enjoyed his fourth), I was highly inebriated and feeling very amorous. It felt cathartic and freeing to express long overdue love for the man who patiently and calmly walked beside me through the fires of infertility and would surely be a kind and compassionate future father to our adopted child.

For the past several years, romance had been gathering dust in a corner due to menstrual cycle charts, thermometers, ovulation sticks, and then fertility drug schedules. In the mad pursuit of pregnancy and parenthood, date nights ceased to exist, foreplay wasn't a priority, and sex became mechanical. Being intimate was no longer euphoric or even mildly pleasurable; it had become an exhausting and stressful chore, filled with unachieved expectations and regular disappointments.

There were countless occasions (let's just say four solid years) when the timing was right, but the mood wasn't. Depression, miscarriages, and fertility treatments had taken their toll on my body; I didn't feel sexy, I felt bloated. My breasts may have grown porn star huge, but I swear it hurt when my husband simply looked at them, let alone tried to touch them. Plus, my hips and abdomen were covered with bruises from countless fertility drug injections. I was perpetually nauseous and felt like throwing up during sex, and a variety of doctors invaded my nether regions on a much too frequent basis. We tried watching porn, but while it provided some comic relief, it left us feeling more dejected and frustrated. We weren't permitted to get liquored up, and I wouldn't even allow myself chocolate.

We were committed to each other and our marriage, but we were in trouble. Infertility had sapped the life out of our relationship and weakened the strength of our love.

While in China, I finally let go of several tons of stress, guilt, and anxiety. I also released myself from the crushing weight of constantly questioning who was at fault for our infertility and placing the burden of guilt upon myself.

For the first time in years, I felt present in my relationship with my husband and thankful for the many gifts of my marriage. I realized that I wasn't alone in my suffering, he had been through hell too and was still by my side. I needed to appreciate him and longed to re-bond with him.

Maybe it was the contagious energy of China or the new and often bizarre sights, sounds, and tastes. Possibly it was the anonymity of hotel rooms or our frequent sampling of Chinese liquor. Maybe it was simply being in a completely different environment, miles away from the pain and suffering at home. Whatever the reasons, I felt alive, I felt naturally amorous, and I felt in love again.

I came to realize, if we were to survive this battle, we needed
to treat each other as equals, work as a team, and remember to
show each other compassion. In the end, it didn't matter how or
why we found ourselves in an infertile situation. All that mattered
was that we were in it together, and the key to survival was the
strength of our commitment, determination, and love.

⚘

While the Big Banyan Tree seemed to have inspired a day
and evening of romance for Chris and me, it is not China's only
nod to true love. In a land filled with ancient traditions, it's no
surprise that the Chinese have a festival in celebration of romance.
On the seventh day of the seventh lunar month, the Chinese
honor the clandestine lovers the Cowherd and the Weaving
Maiden. The festival has a ridiculous number of names including
the Qixi, Qiqiao, Double Seventh and Magpie Festival, as well as
Chinese Valentine's Day. No matter the name, the day is a time to
celebrate true love and wish for a happy marriage and the blessing
of children.

Based on Chinese folklore, the Weaving Maiden was the
seventh daughter of the Sun God of Heaven. Upon visiting earth,
she fell in love with a handsome cowherd. They married and
lived happily on earth, until the Gods became angered that the
cowherd was neglecting his livestock and the maiden ceased her
needlework (some say she weaved beautiful clouds).

The maiden was forced to return to the heavens, and when
the cowherd attempted to follow her, the Heavenly Mother waved
her silver hairpin to create a river of stars too wide to cross (the
Milky Way). One night a year, on the seventh day of the seventh
lunar month, if the skies are clear, magpies form a bridge over

the silver river, so the lovers can reunite. Should it rain and the magpies are unable to gather, the couple's tears fall as rain until they meet again. From what I experienced, it rains a lot in China, with areas of southern China averaging ten to sixteen days of rain during the seventh lunar month, so I wish the ill-fated lovers the best of luck!

With the exception of a single night, the couple lives in separate constellations: The Cowherd as the star Altair in the Aquila constellation and the Weaving Maiden is Vega in the Lyra constellation—two stars separated by the Milky Way.

Traditionally, the Double Seventh Festival is a day of seeking fortunes and reading omens, as well as displaying one's domestic skills and competing in sewing contests. In old China, a woman's sewing ability was highly revered and her worth was determined by the quality of her needlework.

"On the evening of Double Seventh, women traditionally gathered together to honor the celestial Seven Sisters and ask for a good spouse, happy marriage, and many children," Claire told us. "Altars were prepared with the finest needlework, cosmetics and beauty products, and seven plates of food."

In ancient China, not only would I have been cast out for my infertility, I would have been considered worthless for my lack of domestic skills since I can neither cook nor sew. Chris took home-economics in middle and high school and is therefore officially in charge of all sewing related household projects, as well as all electrical, automotive, and technical concerns—and he does our taxes. Just about all I'm good for is my anal-retentive organization skills, my ability to turn a phrase, and a flair for anything creative—other than needlework.

Long ago, a maiden's sewing skills could be foretold by reading the shadows of floating needles. If the shadow cast by a needle on a bowl of water looked like a flower, the maiden would be a skilled seamstress. However, if the shadow was thin like a stick, she should seek work in the kitchen. (I'm guessing my needle would have sunk.) Another way they predicted a maiden's sewing abilities was with spider boxes. Spiders were placed in boxes on the night of the festival. In the morning if the spider had created a beautiful web, it was a lucky omen for the budding seamstress. (My spider likely would have escaped.)

Sadly, many of the ancient customs surrounding Double Seventh Day have been long forgotten and replaced with modern, Western, Valentine's Day traditions like celebrating with red roses, chocolates, and fancy dinners. (It just doesn't have the same charm as fortune telling spiders.)

Still many modern Chinese women pray to the Weaving Maiden on Double Seventh Day. In addition to the patron saint of needlework and the home, the Weaving Maiden is believed to be the protector of orphaned girls and possesses great compassion for the plight of all young women.

While I barely possess the ability to sew on a button, I hoped creating an altar for the heavenly Seven Sisters and wishing for clear skies on Double Seventh Day would protect my little orphaned girl, endear my plea for motherhood to the heavens, and finally unite us with our destined child.

That evening, we watched the mind-blowing Liu Sanjie Impression Light Show created by Zhang Yi Mou, the director and choreographer of the opening ceremony for the 2008 Olympics in Beijing and several movies including *Raise the Red*

Lantern. And yes, it was the same lovestruck, Zhuang minority songstress who professed her love under the Big Banyan Tree.

The stunning scenery of Yangshuo formed what was claimed to be the largest natural, outdoor theater in the world, seating three thousand. The sparkling waters of the Li River set the stage and a dozen beautifully lit karst hills formed a backdrop. Meanwhile, more than six hundred locals, including farmers, fisherman, and young students mainly from the Zhuang minority, sang and danced on top of small, flat rafts and canoes. Rain, mist and moonlight, together with numerous stage lights and fog machines, created a magical effect. The performers appeared to simply float across the water.

The show was about a beautiful, young woman named Liu Sanjie (Third Sister Liu). She had a voice like an angel and was in love with a village farm boy. However, an evil warlord was smitten with her and stole her away. The farm boy and the villagers rallied together to free her, and everyone lived happily ever after—at least I'm pretty sure that 'as the gist of the story.

Hundreds of performers waved lanterns and torches, rippled long, red ribbons and twirled red umbrellas in rhythmic unison. The actors glided around on tiny, invisible rafts and atop underwater walkways (even a few farm animals braved "open" water). The lit-up performers and stage props created intricate designs throughout the dark water.

The grand finale involved a dancer dressed all in white gliding out into the middle of the water on top of a barge with a large, crescent moon.

The dancer told the story of the Moon Goddess, Chang'e in Mandarin and Chang'o or Shang'o in Cantonese. According to legend, thousands of years ago there were ten suns in the sky. The suns burnt all the plants, and the people were dying until an excellent archer named Hou Yi shot down nine of the suns, leaving one to nourish and warm the earth. The Queen of Heaven named Hou Yi the Divine Archer, Ruler of the Solar System and gave him a bottle of elixir that could render a single person immortal. He chose to remain with his wife, Chang'e, and simply kept the potion. One day while Hou Yi was away, his archery student, Pang Meng, tried to steal the elixir. Afraid for her life, Chang'e decided to drink the elixir, which caused her to fly to the moon, where she forever remains, together with a jade rabbit and a woodcutter.

Chinese children are taught to believe that Chang'e still lives on the moon. While fascinating, I fail to see the educational component to this story for children. Try as I might, I can't quite grasp its moral. Don't leave potions of immortality lying around the house? Drinking an elixir to stop a thief is not the best solution? When drinking a potion for long life leave some for your husband?

A second version of this tale claims that fame corrupted Hou Yi, and he became an oppressive tyrant, leading Chang'e to drink the elixir out of desperation. I suppose this rendition has a bit more of a plausible moral element. Don't let fame go to your head and treat your wife well or she might fly away to the moon, literally.

Either way, a devastated Hou Yi built his wife a Moon Palace with an altar filled with her favorite foods among a grove of cinnamon trees. On the fifteenth day of each lunar month, the heavens permit the Divine Archer and Chang'e to reunite under the light of a full moon. Today, believers make offerings to Chang'e in hopes of peace and good luck and look for her image in the bright, full moon (something I planned to do, when and if it ever stopped raining).

As much as we enjoyed our overnight trip to Yangshuo, the Yangshuo Paradise Hotel was not the paradise we had hoped for. I'm guessing that the family staying in the room directly above us managed to squeeze upwards of a dozen family members, including cranky grandma, surely teenagers, wild toddlers, and crying babies into one room. They sounded like a combination of a Chinese adaptation of the *Jerry Springer Show* and a herd of rhinos stomping out a fire. After a night spent listening to a baby scream as if all its milk turned to lemonade, we awoke to a view of an enormous, two-story McDonald's, which was the only thing visible in the pouring rain.

Our return trip to Guilin sadly involved an hour-and-a-half-long taxi ride, since the charming four-hour river cruise to Yangshuo is only available downstream. We had to cancel our plan to stop at the Shangri-La Park (a Chinese version of Disneyland with a boat ride, cave tour, and minority song and dance performances) due to the weather. While I assumed the park would be expensive, crowded, and a bit contrived, I was still disappointed to miss Chinese La-La-Land.

When we first arrived in Guilin, Claire informed us that she asks each of her tour groups to share an expression or urban phrase from their homeland. I had thought long and hard about this important assignment but was completely flummoxed for days. At the end of our trip to Yangshuo, as we were getting out of the taxi in front of our hotel, I spontaneously hollered, "See you later, alligator," and was stunned when Claire responded, "In a while, crocodile." Damn! Some other random traveler had beat me to it. So the next morning, when Claire met us to take us to the airport, I asked, "What's up, chicken butt?"

We were sorry to leave our southern Chinese hamlet and wonderful tour guide. We would have happily stayed several more days, soaking up the bewitching, romantic charm of Yangshuo and Guilin, even in the rain. Thanks to the spring weather, we never got our bike ride through the countryside of Yangshuo, nor did we get to experience the Yulong River by precarious bamboo raft. Sadly, I never did see a dragon, although I'm convinced they were hiding in the mist.

I hope to be fortunate enough to return to China someday with my daughter, at which point we will head to the Guangxi region to continue my search for dragons. Surely together, luck will be on our side, and we will spot one of these wonderous creatures and share some magical memories.

8

MOONCAKES AND TEA

Based on an old Chinese belief, a person's good fortune is directly linked to the happiness of his or her ancestral spirits, and that the departed rule over nature and destiny. Therefore, for centuries, the Qing Ming Festival has been a time for the living to care for the dead and in return receive a bountiful harvest and luck-filled year.

Our flight to Hangzhou on China Southern Airlines was completely packed since it was two days before the Qing Ming or Clear Brightness Festival, which is from April 4 to April 6, or 106 days after the winter solstice. Millions of Chinese were traveling to visit family and the graves of their ancestors—and we were right in the middle of it. Indeed, our plane smelled like a florist shop due to the vast number of passengers carrying large bouquets of colorful flowers.

Honoring the dearly departed during Qing Ming involves four steps. First, all the winter debris must be cleared from the gravesites and replaced by bouquets of spring flowers. Next, offerings of favorite foods and drinks, like tea and alcohol, are made (and all liquids must be poured into the ground, so the ancestors can fully enjoy the gift). Next, a pair of red candles is lit and joss paper, also known as spirit money offerings (ornately decorated paper that ensures the deceased have access to good things in the afterlife) are burnt to complete ash, so they can rise to heaven. Lastly, family members form a line and then one by one they show their respect by bowing three times to the grave, while holding three lit sticks of incense in both hands.

In addition, during this time many Chinese begin their spring planting, set off fireworks to frighten evil spirits, and celebrate by flying kites. Since the willow tree grows in all climates, it is a symbol of vitality in a time of darkness; therefore, many Chinese decorate their homes and persons with willow branches to ward off any evil spirits harboring a grudge that may return during the festival.

The Qing Ming Festival reminded me of growing up in New Mexico and celebrating Dia de los Muertos or Day of the Dead in early November. The holiday originated in Mexico and also is based on remembering ancestors, celebrating with family, and creating *ofrendas* or altars. However, the Latin American version has a flare for the macabre with dancing *calacas* (skeletons), *pan de muerto* (bread of the dead), and sugar skulls. It's a straight up party with lots of revelry, costumes, and tequila.

The official flower of the Day of the Dead is the marigold, since the yellow and orange flowers are thought to guide spirits to their altars via their bright color and strong smell, along with the light from millions of candles.

Qing Ming is one of many festivals honoring the dead in China. During the Hungry Ghost Festival, the gates of the underworld are said to open on the fifteenth day of the seventh month, allowing the hungry ghosts to roam the earth. They live in a continual state of limbo, having been victims of unfortunate or premature death.

To pacify these forgotten souls and prevent them from wreaking havoc, simple offerings are placed in public areas, alongside highways and at intersections, but never at home. All boats are anchored, no fish are caught, and lantern boats are set sail. People visit temples to say a prayer and burn incense and joss paper for the lost, hungry souls.

In a country experiencing extremely rapid modernization, economic growth, and social change, historic festivals such as the Qing Ming Festival help keep modern Chinese citizens connected to their country's past, their ancestors, and their ancient traditions. Since the chaos and intense energy of modern China can be a bit overwhelming, it was refreshing to observe old-world traditions still being celebrated. Having observed the rapid deterioration of culture in my own country, I have a lot of admiration for the Chinese and their ability to balance modern life with ancient tradition and wisdom. Seeing all the Chinese traveling to honor their ancestors made me realize that I've never once visited the graves of my grandparents (but I do light candles for them, occasionally, when I remember).

Hangzhou's two major industries and claims to fame are plant nurseries and tea plantations.

Hangzhou is revered in China for being the only place where the famed Longjing or Dragon Well Green Tea is grown. The city is also praised for its many plant nurseries filled with decorative trees, such as bonsai trees, and fruit trees and for providing all the trees for the Beijing Olympics. During the Song dynasty from 1138 to 1279, Hangzhou was the southern capital of China. Marco Polo referred to Hangzhou as the "city of heaven" and "the finest and most splendid city in all the world."

According to our new guide, Ricky, who was friendly, talkative, and surprisingly tall, the color of Hangzhou is green for its trees. Beijing's color is yellow due to the desert sand and the favorite royal color of its emperors. Suzhou (our next destination) is pink in honor of the local silk industry and Shanghai (our final destination) is gray due to its many skyscrapers.

In addition to a color, most cities in China have their own city god. The city god of Hangzhou is Zhou Chu. Ricky informed us that the ancient temple of Zhou Chu had become a very expensive teahouse, which served three-hundred-yuan (forty-seven-dollar)-per-cup Longjing green tea.

In Hangzhou, we stayed at the Lakeview Hotel; a modern, high-rise on the banks of the West Lake. While there are thirty-six lakes in China named West Lake, Hangzhou's West Lake, or Xi Hú, is by far the most famous.

Many legends surround West Lake, the most famous of which tells the love story of Bai Suzhen and Xu Xian. Long ago, two snakes, one green and one white, meditated for years until they turned into beautiful women. Every day, the sisters enjoyed basking in the sun. One day, the white snake spirit, Bai Suzhen, met a handsome boy named Xu Xian. They fell in love and married. But an old monk named Fa Hai thought it indecent for a human and an animal to marry, so he forced them to separate (some say he tricked Bai Suzhen into drinking an elixir that revealed her true form and repelled Xu Xian). Xu Xian died of sadness, the white lady was imprisoned under the Leifeng Pagoda, and the green lady disappeared. Another more optimistic version of the tale claims that the green lady, Xiao Qing, rescued the couple and they lived happily ever after.

Near the Xīlíng Bridge is the tomb of fifth-century courtesan and poet Su Xiaoxiao. She died at the age of nineteen due to illness, but some say she died from grief awaiting the return of her lover and now haunts the island. Many have claimed to hear the sound of tinkling bells on the gown of Su Xiaoxiao as her spirit wanders around West Lake at night.

Regardless of its tragic or happy endings, West Lake is now a hot spot for new couples, date nights, and weddings. It would be hard not to be in a romantic mood in such a charming setting, and Chris and I fell deeply under its magical spell.

One afternoon we took a short cruise around West Lake on a boat with an enormous golden dragon head and tail and two sitting pavilions in the middle. We traveled to one of three islands on the lake. Paradise Island (or Donut Island, as Ricky called it) consists of a ring of land in the middle of the West Lake. This island is bisected twice by two bridges to form a cross. A ghost busting, zigzag bridge, known as a nine-turn bridge, leads to a teahouse named Heart Linked to Heart Pavilion. No tea party crashing ghosts allowed!

The island is also home to Flower and Harbor Park, which was in full bloom with pink and white plum and cherry blossoms, bushes with bright yellow flowers, and weeping willow trees hanging down into the water. Winding paths bordered by large flat rocks that doubled as seats lined the lake's edge. In the distance, tall pagodas topped the many lush hills and various ornate tour boats, and small fishing crafts dotted the lake. It was serene, bordering on heavenly.

Paradise Island is best known for the Three Pools Mirroring the Moon display. The "Three Pools" refer to the three stone pagodas placed at the vertexes of a triangle in the deepest water (nearly ten feet deep) off the shore of the island. The towers feature an empty sphere with six evenly distributed holes. During full moons, candles are placed inside the spheres, and the holes are covered with thin paper. The stunning effect is that of multiple full moons reflecting on the water. The Three Pools Mirroring the Moon is featured on the back of the one-yuan bill.

During the Moon Festival, people gather at Three Pools Mirroring the Moon on Paradise Island in West Lake to drink tea, eat moon cakes, and watch the "moons" glow.

There is no shortage of festivals in China. The Moon Festival, or Mid-Autumn Festival, is the second grandest festival in China, after Chinese New Year. Falling on the fifteenth day of the eighth month, based on the Chinese lunar calendar, it is celebrated when the moon is at its roundest and brightest.

The ancient Chinese observed that the moon's movements are closely tied to the changes of seasons. Hence, to express their gratitude to the moon and celebrate the harvest season, they offer gifts and thanks during the festival. The full moon symbolizes the connection between past, present, and future and the cycle of life.

The Moon Festival wouldn't be complete without moon cakes (*yuebing*). The round cakes have a wheat flour outer shell—which is often stamped with a beautiful flower, scroll design, or Chinese character—while the inside has a dense filling of lotus seed, winter melon, green tea, or sweet red bean paste (or in more modern times, chocolate or ice cream). The center is often filled with a whole duck egg, which represents the full moon, and is considered very lucky.

My first taste of authentic moon cakes was during a walking tour of Chinatown on a trip to San Francisco, ten months after getting on the adoption waiting list. Chris and I ate dumplings and moon cakes, visited a teahouse, pharmacy, and fortune cookie factory and got a mah-jongg lesson from some friendly seniors in a park. Upon visiting a Buddhist temple, a monk gave me a small, fabric prayer square on a red cord, which I wore wrapped around my wrist (until it began to disintegrate, so I placed it on my fertility altar next to my statue of the Laughing Buddha).

In my opinion, moon cakes are almost too ornate to eat. It's not easy taking a big bite out of a moon cake's lovely, decorative shell. Red bean paste is the most traditional filling but a bit of an acquired taste. I didn't care for it at first but have grown to love it, since sweet red bean paste is the main ingredient in numerous Chinese delicacies.

Moon cakes are extremely dense; just one bite can quell a craving for sweets and a whole one is a complete meal (well maybe not by American standards, but let's just say, moon cakes are filling). Moon cakes aren't simply round, beautiful, and delicious, they are also a valuable part of China's history. Moon cakes were instrumental in the overthrow of the Mongolian ruled Yuan dynasty since they were used to distribute secret messages (like a less obvious fortune cookie).

During the Moon Festival, the time for paying homage to the moon is after dinner. A table is placed outdoors with an offering of thirteen moon cakes stacked in a pyramid. A complete lunar year contains thirteen months; therefore, the offering signifies happiness for a full year. The moon cake's roundness symbolizes a complete family circle. I couldn't wait to share a moon cake with my husband and soon-to-be daughter at the massive Mid-Autumn Festival celebration sponsored by our adoption agency.

The Chinese also eat other round foods during the festival including gourds (for togetherness), apples (sounds like "peace"), peaches (for longevity), pears and grapes (since they are round like the moon), as well as pomegranates and watermelon (whose seeds symbolize many children). At the height of the full moon, families snack on lucky foods, decorate with paper lanterns, and share their secrets and dreams with Chang'e, the Moon Goddess—in hopes their wishes will come true.

According to Ricky there is a saying that Hangzhou is the capital of tea in China and Longjing tea is the best. Therefore, while in Hangzhou, we visited the village of Meijiawu, one of the only places in China where Dragon Well green tea is grown.

Tea is a five-thousand-year-old cultural tradition and art form in China. Some believe Buddhism may have played a role in the Chinese love of tea. As the story goes the monk Bodhidharma, a master of meditation, vowed to sit nine straight years in a cave outside Nanjing. As the days passed and his task grew more difficult, according to legend, the first tea seedlings sprouted from his eyelashes as a helpful aid to staying alert while meditating.

The picturesque village of Meijiawu consists of small white houses; farmers in wide-brimmed, pointed straw hats; and neatly planted rows of tea bushes in lines across the hills. The hillsides in spring literally glow a bright, fresh green. The organized rows of tea bushes were reminiscent of the terraced rice fields but taller, thicker, and basically bushier.

According to Ricky, all of the female residents of the poor farming community turned wealthy tea growing village have the first name of Mei and men are considered lucky if they marry a Mei Girl. Just one more reason why I liked the name Mei for our future daughter.

There are six types of Chinese tea that originate from the Camellia Sinensis plant. Each tastes uniquely different based on varied processing and fermenting techniques. Green tea, by far the most popular, is immediately dried to avoid oxidation and then heated to prevent fermentation. Hong Cha, which literally means "red tea" but Westerners call black tea is fermented and fully oxidized for a strong and hearty flavor. Oolong or Black Dragon tea, which is unique to China, is a partially fermented option that's less astringent than green tea but milder than black. Pu-erh tea is an exotic and earthy fermented tea from Yunnan province, which traditionally comes in bricks or flat cakes. White tea is a rare, sun-dried, light and smooth alternative to green, black, and oolong. Lastly, aromatized, flavored tea combines tea leaves with flowers or fruit essence, the most beloved and popular of which is fragrant jasmine tea.

In Meijiawu the Mei women pick the tea (because they have patience), while the men dry and then stir-fry the tea in tea seed oil. The Chinese drink green tea in summer to clear out heat in the blood and black tea in the winter to warm the stomach. The village has roughly 160 teahouses run by local families, possibly due to the Chinese saying, "It is better to live three days without salt than one day without tea."

We learned that there are many hard rules and traditional customs when it comes to drinking tea in China. Our Chinese tea etiquette lessons were held at a large Longjing teahouse, factory, and sales room. The stately courtyard featured a lovely fountain consisting of a huge earthen teapot pouring water into an oddly milky, pastel-blue pond filled with giant, colorful koi fish. There was also a statue of the tea god, Lu Yu, pleasant sitting areas, and numerous decorative bonsai trees.

We were presented with various types of loose green tea in flat, woven bamboo trays and spent over an hour drinking and learning about different qualities of green tea. Dried orange rinds were used to sweeten the tea (and supposedly increase blood circulation). We were also given a demonstration on how green tea can clear iodine from a bowl of rice; the water turned from brown to purple to clear.

Chinese tea etiquette dictates that you are not to fill your own teacup. Instead you are to attend only to your neighbor's cup and in return your neighbor will attend to yours. (Filling your own cup implies your neighbor was shamefully negligent.) If you are served a half cup of tea, it indicates that your host welcomes you and is not busy. However, if you are served a full cup of tea, you had best drink it quickly and get going, because your host has no time to chat. Be careful to never point the spout of a teapot toward anyone, as it is considered impolite. If you tap the table three times with two fingers while having tea, it means thank you very much.

Longjing tea leaves are picked four times per year. The best Mingqian tea is harvested in the spring during the Qing Ming Festival (unplanned, perfect timing on our part). Lesser quality and significantly cheaper forms of the green tea are produced in the summer and fall.

A half kilo of the best, spring, Mingqian tea sells for 3,000 yuan ($473) for roughly 300 cups of tea. I'm embarrassed to admit, we got caught up in the spring harvest and Qing Ming festival excitement and spent nearly $100 on tea (and I honestly can't tell the difference between Hangzhou's legendary Dragon Well and Colorado's own Celestial Seasonings green tea). The highest quality tea came in small, red tins with gold lettering and images of happy, playful children. The lesser quality, "swag tea" came in brown tins with a lovely landscape image of mountains shrouded in mist.

According to the purveyors of tea, green tea is an excellent antioxidant for overall cleansing. The steam from a hot cup of green tea is good for dry eyes. Also, green tea contains fluoride, reduces high blood pressure, and decreases the oils in fats to assist in weight loss (or so the charming saleswoman claimed).

I'm likely to remain a serious coffee addict for life, but thanks to my trip to China and learning about the many health benefits of green tea, I have a new appreciation for the herbal caffeine fix. I began chugging antioxidant-rich green tea leading up to any baby-making efforts in hopes of purification (mostly of my coffee addiction). Now I temper my borderline insane consumption of coffee with occasional cups of green tea for variety. And if it's true that green tea promotes weight loss, who wouldn't want to lose a few pounds?

During the ride back to Hangzhou, I was greatly intrigued by a bumper sticker I saw on the back of a sedan featuring a female stick figure sitting in a chair. Ricky explained that the "mommy in a chair" bumper sticker equated to the American "baby on board" sticker.

Seeing the rather strange, Chinese family pride sticker made me think of the many dejecting days, when I had pulled up behind a minivan with a row of stickers—Disney ears, zombies, machine guns or flip flops—representing family members. Several years of failed pregnancy attempts, stressful fertility treatments, and heartbreaking miscarriages had made me seriously jealous and frighteningly crazy! So much so that there might have been a rear ending.

Sometimes with infertility it was easy to feel like a remote island, alone at sea while everyone else was anchored to their families. But almost every woman has a story about pregnancy or child loss, whether her own or someone she loves, but sadly many stories go unshared, many misfortunes are hidden, and too many women suffer in silence. Maybe it's our rugged individualism, but Americans seem to have few support systems or recovery rituals for healing from miscarriage, stillbirth, or the death of a child. Many women hide pregnancy losses and conceal their shame over feeling faulty (even though it's estimated that one out of three or roughly 33 percent of known pregnancies end in miscarriage).

My mother suffered a stillborn, what would have been my (second) older brother and my mother's first child, and it took her seven years to have a child—me. In the late sixties and early seventies, the doctors' best guess as to the culprit behind the many fruitless years was my father's liquor habit. Her unbearable loss, long journey, and unwavering strength helped to lessen the magnitude of my own infertility by showing me I wasn't singularly cursed or alone in my misery. Her story helped me to keep my personal hardships in perspective to the long suffering of women throughout the world.

In Asia, they not only have a deity dedicated to protecting the souls of lost children, there's also a therapeutic grieving ceremony for child loss. Revered in East Asian Buddhism and often depicted as a Buddhist monk, Jizō's Sanskrit name, Ksitigarbha, translates to "Earth Womb." In many cultures, he is regarded as the bodhisattva of the underworld, but in Japan he is one of the most beloved deities and the guardian of *misuko* or children lost to miscarriage, stillbirth, or an early death.

In Japanese mythology, the souls of children who died before their parents are unable to cross the mythical Sanzu River to the afterlife because they have not had enough time to accumulate good deeds and left their parents in anguish. It is believed that

Jizō saves these poor souls from having to pile stones along the bank of the river for eternity as penance. Instead, he hides the children in his robe, recites mantras, and assists them through reincarnation.

During a *mizuko kuyō* (offering to water children) ceremony, the Japanese pile stones at the base of Jizō statues to shorten the time their lost child must suffer in the underworld or endure an illness. The statues are often decorated with children's clothes and covered with offerings of toys, food, flowers, candles, incense, and written prayers.

I learned about Jizō after my second miscarriage, which required an emotionally traumatic surgery to remove the non-viable fetus. After the surgery, I placed a Ksitigarbha figurine carved out of a small, black stone and with a serene face, closed eyes, and hands clasped in prayer upon an altar. The statue looked part holy monk and part innocent child. I added sonogram photos and an engraved silver rattle from my childhood to honor and protect my lost child. It helped me to believe my *mizuko* was being cared for and to bid the child a final farewell and wish my baby luck in its next life.

I'm proud to say that Chris and I braved the famous Zhiweiguan restaurant all by ourselves. The walk-up, street-corner restaurant looked extremely popular based on the crowd of about forty locals around the glass display counters impatiently shouting out orders and waving their hands in the air, in typical Chinese fashion. After pacing back and forth several times perusing the options, looking for a next-in-line ticket dispenser, and making eyes at the servers, it became clear that no one planned to take our order in a civilized manner. It was complete anarchy, and the English-speaking Americans were getting nowhere. We were going to have to get down and dirty, Chinese-style.

That's when we decided I must use my long-blonde hair to stand out from the crowd. I'm not proud of my tactics, but if you want to get anywhere in China, you must act like a local, throw caution (and manners) to the wind, and jump headfirst into chaos. We needed to gain an advantage, so I took off my baseball cap, started swinging my hair around, and almost immediately a server motioned to me. Game. Set. Match. We got served!

After successfully getting the male server's attention, I started smiling and pointing at random, unknown meal options. I pointed to tempura chicken (which I had hoped was going to be vegetables); tofu (which as much as I normally enjoy tofu had a weird slimy consistency in China); marinated vegetables (which had too much vinegar and were gross); a duck leg (for Chris which he said was dry); a thin pancake filled with greens (which constituted my main meal); and a sesame bun filled with potatoes, onions, and ham (which to my surprise I also liked, but had to share with Chris). For dessert, I pointed at sesame balls filled with a sweet red bean paste which tasted like strawberry BBQ sauce. We both loved them and wished we had gotten more but decided it wasn't worth waging a second hair waving assault.

We felt very proud of ourselves for fighting through a mob of locals to obtain our take-out street food like total ninja badasses using the ancient "hair flip and point" technique. The huge amount of food cost forty-six yuan or less than eight dollars. While enjoying the spoils of battle, we scanned through the channels on the hotel television, searching for something remotely understandable. We ended up watching mostly Chinese commercials—95 percent of which were for mysterious medications and the rest advertised miracle face creams.

While visiting the Qinghefang Ancient Street, I believe I discovered the driving force behind China's booming economy: the red lantern industry. It appeared every inch of the massive country of China was covered in red lanterns, nowhere more so than the Qinghefang Ancient Street. The two-story, white buildings with ornate dark woodwork, antique wrought-iron lampposts, and towering trees nestled along the ancient street turned modern pedestrian mall were completely plastered with red lanterns, tassels, and banners.

The street was at the heart of old Hangzhou and was a former center of politics, culture, and commerce in the ancient city. During the Southern Song dynasty from 1127 to 1279 AD, the street was lined with shops, restaurants, and teahouses. While Qinghefang Street had become a major tourist attraction and pedestrian shopping mall, many authentic, century-old shops hide among the giant souvenir stores, perfume and cosmetics boutiques, and trendy clothing stores.

According to Ricky, the outdoor mall was carefully restored as an exact copy of an eight-hundred-year-old painting of Qinghefang Street during the Qing Ming Festival. The street did indeed look very old, authentic, and festive, even with throngs of tourists talking on cell phones while clutching white plastic bags filled with gaudy souvenirs.

We visited a tiny, narrow (the width of Chris and I holding hands and stretching our arms to the sides) shop featuring rows upon rows of Chinese fans. The ceiling of the already cluttered store was covered with open, upside-down, waxed-paper umbrellas. We had to duck down to avoid becoming impaled. At five eight, I'm generally considered slightly tall for a woman in the States; but in China, I felt like a freakishly tall, stunningly pale, and noticeably blonde giantess.

Meanwhile, Chris, who is also five eight but with brown hair and eyes and olive skin, has the uncanny ability to blend into any environment. While in Costa Rica, the Ticos thought he was a native, and he fit right in with the locals while in Turkey and Greece. Plus, he has a natural gift with languages, having taught himself Swedish, simply because he likes the people, culture, and country. While he would never be mistaken for Chinese, at least he didn't stick out like a porcupine at a nudist colony.

9

BODY AND SOUL

While traveling through China, it was easy to get temple fever, in the same way that tourists in Europe get overwhelmed by the number of cathedrals and visitors to Mexico and Central America burn out on seeing ancient Mayan ruins. Eventually, the expression "seen one, seen them all" holds true. Not so, with the Lingyin Temple and surrounding Feilai Feng Buddhist scenic area, for it was truly extraordinary and left a lasting impression.

As I struggled to find inspiration and hope, I felt a real connection with the Lingyin Temple or Temple of Soul's Retreat. The largest Buddhist temple and monastery in the Wulin Mountains of Southern China was surrounded by forested hills on three sides and got its name due to its tranquil setting (at a time when silent monks were the only residents, not hordes of disquieting tourists, but still the site was divine).

The Buddhist center was founded in AD 328 during the Eastern Jin dynasty by an Indian monk and from its inception was the pride of the Zhejiang Province. At its peak, the complex featured nine multi-story buildings, eighteen pavilions, seventy-two halls, thirteen hundred dormitory rooms and was inhabited by more than three thousand monks.

In addition to the Four Heavenly Guardians, we learned that in every Buddhist temple, the first hall must prominently feature a happy Buddha. At Lingyin Temple, the entrance hall displayed the main incarnation of Maitreya Buddha, more commonly known as the Laughing Buddha. It is said he could endure all intolerance due to his good and loving character and that he is always fat, happy, and smiling. The most ancient and important statue featured throughout the complex is that of Skanda Buddha or Wei Tuo in Chinese, who is charged with guarding the teachings of Buddhism.

I noticed a symbol on a Buddha's chest, which looked exactly like a Nazi swastika, only backwards. To my surprise, I learned the name swastika comes from Sanskrit and means well-being or good luck. According to Ricky, in Buddhism the geometrical figure is very fortuitous as it symbolizes the footprints of Buddha, which represent the power of life. Regardless of what I learned, it was still highly unnerving to see commonality between two such different philosophies and historical movements.

At Lingyin Temple, we were told a rather brief story of the creation of Buddhism and history of Sakayamuni. According to Ricky, Sakayamuni went into the jungle where a deer gave him milk and the monkeys gave him food for seven days and nights; afterward he reached enlightenment—if only it was that easy!

Ricky's version was certainly more succinct and realistic than the creation story carved with gems on a wall of the Da Ci'en Temple in Xi'an. However, I couldn't help but wonder if Ricky gave us the condensed version for tourists and skipped a few rather important parts.

Throughout the temple complex, magnificently detailed and realistic carved dragons wrapped around the different tiers of the temples and appeared to fly out from under the eaves. Tiny cast-iron bells hung from the very tips of the eaves, as though the dragons were reaching for them. The incredibly lifelike dragon statues had raised scales, rows of pointed teeth, and ridiculously long whiskers. The dragons were truly breathtaking, but few people were likely to notice them—unless they looked up toward the heavens.

If any place were to help me believe in the power of religion, it would be the Feilai Feng Buddhist park. It was truly humbling and inspiring to witness the many Buddhist inscriptions and effigies painstakingly created by generations of ardent believers. The works of art throughout the grounds of the monastery were true examples of sincere devotion, faith, and love.

Feilai Feng means the "peak flown from afar," the "peak that flew hither," or simply "flying peak" and got its many names because the peak is limestone while the surrounding hills are sandstone; therefore, it was said the peak flew from a distant land. Many believe the hill was originally from India but flew to Hangzhou overnight as a demonstration of the omnipotence of Buddhism.

We walked along a rather precarious and slippery path to view the many rock reliefs that dot the face of the craggy peak. We also discovered numerous carvings of Buddhas hidden in caves and grottoes. A wide variety of plaques and statues were stacked on top of each other, sometimes covering the rocky face of Flying Peak from top to bottom, three to four carvings deep.

A happy Buddha sat within a small round cave, while a tall, thin statue of Guanyin (Goddess of Mercy) was carved into the rock directly above. Moss-covered stairs led adventurous visitors to a large oblong cave filled with a rather rotund Buddha statue surrounded by at least a dozen small disciples. A long, narrow carving along the base of the peak depicted a religious pilgrimage on horseback, while a traditional carving of Sakayamuni sitting on top of a lotus bud was etched into the rock face directly above. A small bronze pagoda sat atop a cave filled with a statue of Guanyin with one palm facing downward, while next to it a Buddha wearing a flower crown was missing one hand. Within a large cave dedicated to the bodhisattva Guanyin, a small crack reached to the surface and those standing above the cave could see a sliver of sunlight, known as the "One Thread of Heaven." Of all the incredible carvings, my personal favorite was the enormous statue of a Buddha riding atop an elephant, where each of the elephant's feet rested upon lotus buds.

The more than three hundred statues of Buddhas dated from the tenth to the fourteenth centuries (sadly 40 percent of the Buddhist images were destroyed during the Cultural Revolution). The surrounding rocks were carved with poetry, prayers, and dedications. Thick moss covered the statues and large vines wound around their edges augmenting the passage of time, to create the effect of nature, art, and spirituality becoming one.

There were many traditions to follow while visiting Feilai Feng scenic park for those searching for guidance, hope and a bit of good luck—myself included.

A large statue of Laughing Buddha carried a bag of goods to help the poor, sick, and young. The Laughing Buddha's Chinese name, *Hotei*, means "cloth sack." The buddha's loving character is synonymous with happiness, good luck, and abundance, and he is often surrounded by children. Ricky referred to the happy deity as the Beer Belly Buddha. It is said that rubbing the Laughing Buddha's round belly will bring you luck.

Years ago, before my husband's grandmother left this earth, she gave me a statue of the Laughing Buddha covered in children. Mee Maw Marian spent many years living in Asia and wisely knew the kindhearted deity was exactly what I needed to help me stay positive. Today, this cherished gift is the centerpiece of my collection of Asian folk art, feng shui items, travel mementos, and fertility charms.

At Feilai Feng, a statute of the Buddha of Fortune held a pearl, and it was believed that if you rubbed his foot, he would grant your wish. I closed my eyes, whispered my prayer, and rubbed that Buddha's foot until it shone, in hopes that I would be granted a baby. I was hoping the Buddha of Fortune, in partnership with the Laughing Buddha and the Goddess of Mercy, would together light a symbolic fire under fate's butt.

I was completely enchanted and deeply affected by Feilai Feng park. The way in which the statues and dedications blended into the limestone peak's rocky surface and hid within its caves felt completely holistic, as if the religious nages were part of nature and wondrously belonged there.

I have often wondered if my infertility issues were somehow due to my lack of faith, like symbolic retribution for not believing in a higher power. My home was filled with fertility talismans and religious tokens, yet I actively practiced no religion. I thought of myself as open-minded, maybe even a bit spiritual, but my prayers always felt weak and unsure.

Once, when I was working as a literacy specialist at an elementary school, an unknown parent stopped me in the hallway, informed me that she heard I was doing fertility treatments, and said that God had a plan for me and that I was going against his will. I was completely devastated, had a good cry in the faculty bathroom, then went back to teaching other people's children. But I never recovered from the fear that God's plan was for me to suffer and never become a mother—and not understand why.

While my interest in Buddhism sprang from a desire to connect with the religious history and culture of the country of my future adopted child's birth, my visit to Lingyin Temple left me in a place of true reverence. The Temple of the Soul's Retreat instilled within me a sense of peace and comfort.

I was deeply moved by the artistic expressions of these faithful, bygone Buddhists. No doubt, they spent endless hours hammering away at solid rock, often at perilous heights, to create these beautiful statues, poetic engravings, and other symbols of faith and love. I couldn't fathom the depth of religious belief and devotion that could inspire one to create such magnificent works of art, but I was truly awed and elated. These artists' level of dedication to Buddhism led me to consider my own level of commitment toward starting a family and that maybe funneling that intense energy into religious practice might just be beneficial.

Rebirth is one of the fundamental doctrines of Buddhism. The principal of reincarnation asserts that rebirth is not always in human form, but as existence in one of the six gati, or realms. The realms of rebirth include deva (heavenly), asura (demigod), manusya (human), tiryak (animals), preta (ghost), and naraka (resident of hell). Rebirth is determined by one's karma. Good realms require kushala, or good karma, while a rebirth in an evil realm is a consequence of akushala, or bad karma. Nirvana (a realm free from suffering and endless reincarnation) is the ultimate goal of all Buddhists.

Thanks to China and my exposure to Buddhism, instead of feeling karmically cursed, I felt reborn (or at the very least reawakened). I was moving away from a realm of depression, anxiety, and despair toward a new territory filled with hope, knowledge, and new experiences. My fragile, battered shell of a person was filling up with new energy, passion, and strength. I was a long way from nirvana (or deva and asura for that matter), but my *qi*, or life force, was starting to flow again, and I felt alive for the first time in years.

My soul was awakened and, when it came to my body, I was finding healing there too.

Four years of infertility took a hazardous toll on my physical health. When my body needed help surviving the many side effects of hormone drugs and my mind needed a release from guilt, anxiety, self-criticism, and hopelessness, traditional Chinese medicine (TCM) had been there for me. So after years of beneficial acupuncture treatments in the States, I was excited to learn more about TCM directly from the source.

We learned all about TCM during a visit to the incredible Hu Qing Yu Tang Pharmacy and Museum of Traditional Chinese Medicine on Qinghefang Ancient Street. The pharmacy was opened in 1874 by Hu Xueyan, who was not only a successful businessman but also a high-class official in the imperial court. In China's ancient feudal society, entrepreneurs were looked down upon whereas state officials were highly regarded. The pharmacy, known as the Medicine King south of the Yangtze River, was said to have produced four hundred types of medicine based on secret recipes, proven remedies, and clinical practices.

Not only did the museum, drug store, and living classroom at the Hu Qing Yu Tang Pharmacy offer a fascinating glimpse into

China's long medicinal history, the restored building is a wonder of Chinese architecture. It is two stories and has a central interior courtyard surrounded by a four-sided balcony. It was built from intricately carved dark, cherry wood with painted gold and red accents. The pharmacy could be a set from the hysterical martial arts movie, *The Legend of Drunken Master*, where Jackie Chan plays Wong Fei-Hung, a legendary martial artist, traditional Chinese medicine practitioner, and revolutionary.

Pharmacists in white lab coats and caps climbed up sliding ladders to remove supplies from tiny apothecary boxes, lining the walls from floor to ceiling, to prepare traditional Chinese medications. We learned the Chinese believe scorpion is good for moving stagnant blood; therefore, ground up scorpion is used in many tinctures for treating blood issues.

While we didn't buy any scorpion, snake, or ground antler products, we did purchase a small bottle of white flower analgesic balm, a Chinese, cure-all tincture for ending headaches, relieving stiff muscles, clearing the sinuses, and stopping motion sickness. The tincture is a blend of several essential oils including wintergreen, eucalyptus, peppermint, menthol, camphor, and lavender. With my severe allergies, asthma, and motion sickness, the Chinese cure-all has become a lifesaver (which I now buy in large quantities at the local Asian market and keep small bottles in my purse and car).

I have always been comfortable with alternative, holistic medicine and Eastern medical philosophy since I grew up surrounded by naturopaths, reiki practitioners, believers in rebirthing, acupuncture schools, and super yogis on the West Coast. Meanwhile, Chris is much more skeptical of Eastern medicine and the new-age healing arts. To his credit, he tolerates my mother's use of a pendulum before making all major decisions, so I wasn't going to push the purchase of scorpion powder (but as I found out later, I should have).

After many years of acupuncture treatments, I was no longer phased by nontraditional medical diagnostic questions like "Are you always thirsty?" "Is your skin dry and are your nails brittle?" "Do you have cold feet?" "Are you an insomniac?" "Do you have irregular bowel movements?" "Is your sexual energy low?" To which, I've always answered, yes (to be fair, there's nothing like planned, baby-making sex to decrease your sex drive!).

These questions are always followed by a look at my tongue (which is guaranteed to be cracked and coated in a chalky white film) and a study of my pulse (which is always weak and often erratic). The findings are generally the same: liver qi or energy stagnation.

While Western doctors use the pulse to determine only a heart rate, Eastern pulse diagnosis assesses up to twenty-eight different qualities of one's health. For example, a fast pulse indicates too much heat. Whereas a slow pulse is cold, a strong pulse signals excesses, and a feeble pulse warns of weakness.

Next, my acupuncturist puts tiny, hair-like needles all over my body from the top of my head, center of my forehead, and rim of my right ear to the sides of my wrists, base of my lower belly, inner sides of my calves, and finally between my toes. Most of the time, I feel nothing, but every once in a while, I get a zing of qi. I listen to the gentle sounds of babbling brooks, flamenco guitar, or chanting monks and take a needle nap. Then, I'm sent home smelling like a pine forest with small, square stickers in my ears covering tiny seeds atop calm inducing pressure points.

Through the years, my acupuncturist has become a second mother, offering me endless support and guidance. We have talked for hours and often cried together. She was by my side for each IVF embryo transfer, giving me acupuncture treatments before and after the stressful, clinical process. I would have been lost without her.

While visiting the Hu Qing Yu Tang Pharmacy, I gained many new healing benefits from Chinese medicine. I tried tui na massage, which literally means "pinch and pull" and is not known to be relaxing but rather as a treatment for disharmony. The intense but beneficial massage was paired with cupping, a therapy technique in which heated glass cups are applied to the skin along the meridians of the body, creating suction as a way of stimulating the flow of energy.

I could easily have spent a week at the ancient pharmacy learning, healing, and relaxing, but sadly we were on a tight schedule, with no more time for restorative pursuits (even though they were needed).

According to ancient texts, the sage treats illness before, not after, it has arisen, and he puts his organs in order before they fall into disrepair. Taking medicine to regulate health after you are sick is like digging a well when thirsty or making daggers in the middle of battle.

The first written account of TCM is the *Huangdi Neijing* or *Inner Canon of the Yellow Emperor,* written in the second century BC. The work is composed of two texts, each with eighty-one chapters. They are written in a question-and-answer format between the mythical Yellow Emperor and six of his equally legendary ministers. The first text is called *Suwen* and covers basic questions, fundamentals, and diagnostic methods. The second text, *Lingshu*, reviews acupuncture methods.

Above all else, the Chinese believe that good health depends on the harmony of each organ's yin and yang and that imbalance brings discomfort, pain, and disease. They regard the body as a mass of energy or life force known as *qi*. Therefore, rather than treating targeted areas or organs, Chinese medicine works holistically to maintain yin and yang equilibrium and balanced *qi* throughout the entire body.

The Chinese believe that treatments of illness consist of three stages: healthy diet (medicinal food), physical exercise, and, only as a last resort, medication. Remedies in opposition of the ailment are prescribed to return the body to balance; for example, medications that are hot in nature to treat an illness that is cold in nature.

According to TCM, the key to good health is a calm disposition; excessive emotions, both positive and negative, throw off the body's balance. TCM prescribes avoidance of seven emotions: anger, joy, sadness, grief, stress, fear, and fright. Depression and anger are bad for the liver, while anxiety and sorrow harm the spleen. While these tenets are certainly worthy, achieving such a state is easier said than done. Telling a woman suffering from infertility to keep calm and avoid excessive emotion is ludicrous, preposterous, and damned outrageous!

Due to my infertility, I was already highly knowledgeable of many alternatives to Western medicine. In addition to treatments from my beloved Chinese herbalist and acupuncturist on a regular basis, I tried wearing crystal and magnetized bracelets, drinking fertility boosting tea, and meditating regularly. I had also experimented with salt cave therapy, fertility boosting yoga, hypnosis therapy, and Mayan inner-uterine massage. Yes, that's right, a therapist put her hand up my hoohah to massage my womb in an effort to make it "warm and inviting." Therefore, absolutely nothing about traditional Chinese medicine—from urine, holy water and ant ingestion therapy to being buried in sand or set on fire—phased me in the slightest.

I feel as though I left Hangzhou healed (or at the very least vastly rejuvenated), with heightened physical and mental health, spiritual awareness, and positive energy (not to mention several tins of antioxidant-rich green tea).

This newfound strength and clarity came with a powerful new keepsake.

As we left the Qinghefang Ancient Street shopping area, I found my very own miniature, Chinese turtle-dragon at a cart featuring bonsai trees and garden decor. Throughout our travels, Chris and I had noticed several fascinating statues of a dragon with a turtle shell on guard at museums, palaces, and parks.

According to Ricky, the dragon represents success, power, and courage while the turtle is a symbol for longevity and is often represented carrying the world on its back.

My turtle-dragon guardian is blackened bronze with lovely green accents and mysterious Chinese characters etched into its shell. While I was excited to find a small representation of our beloved turtle-dragon and hoped the powerful memento would give me strength, I was less than thrilled to have to carry the heavy figurine in my backpack. I tried my best to sneak the bronze statue into Chris' backpack, but his tolerance for my many purchases of folk art items, feng shui trinkets, and fertility talismans was wearing thin.

Before leaving Hangzhou, we had one of only a few mediocre meals while in China. My only complaint of our tour experience was the number of lunches at area hotels, since the hotel restaurants always had no atmosphere, bland food and disinterested waitstaff. We both preferred authentically chaotic and colorful local restaurants. However, while the food at the Lilly Hotel was disappointing, it was still a memorable meal, as I made a new friend. I played games over the back of a bench seat with a little Japanese boy. The darling prankster was roughly four years old and would continually pop his head up, flash a huge smile, then disappear in a fit of giggles. Meanwhile, his charming parents smiled and shyly bobbed their heads.

We played several rounds of peek-a-boo and patty-cake, then congratulated each other on our wins with high-fives. Every time he smiled, my uterus, or "lower heart," literally throbbed. As I observed his pure joy, my eyes welled with tears of happiness and pain. It was all I could do not to grab the little cherub and make a run for it.

10

FENG SHUI AND FLOWERS

We surely would have ended up in Inner Mongolia if Ricky hadn't helped us find our three-hour train to Suzhou. He told us about the lights on the digital departure board: orange meant wait, green meant the train was late, blinking red meant board the train, and solid red meant the train was leaving. (It went against every fiber of my American being to board a train with a blinking red light!)

By then we were accustomed to rowdy, uncivilized air travel in China, so we weren't remotely surprised to see children running up and down the center aisle of the moving train. We watched a mother pass out a seven-course breakfast feast to her family across the aisle and over several seats. During the process, brown sauce oozed down the back of a seat, several large gelatinous chunks rolled across the aisle, and an innocent bystander got breakfast all over his shirt.

Travel within the world's most populous country had become so turbulent that in 2014, China began applying a social credit system. Those who had committed a misdeed could be banned from air and train travel for up to a year. The types of social misconduct that could lead to a travel ban spanned from false terrorism threats to causing a disturbance to smoking. In just three years, 6.15 million Chinese citizens were banned from air travel due to inappropriate behavior.

We were left to wonder if the highly intoxicated man sitting two rows in front of us who was chain smoking and yelling at fellow passengers qualified for a travel ban (especially after he threw some sort of bread product at a man who dared to express his disapproval).

Upon disembarking from our train, we were shocked to discover the situation in the train station was equally, if not more, tumultuous. The station in Suzhou was a chaotic free-for-all with hundreds of Chinese trying desperately to be the first to push through one of three turnstiles to freedom. I felt like a grain of sand being pushed by hundreds of other grains of sand toward a ridiculously tiny exit in a proverbial hourglass.

Our new guide, Leo, was waiting for us on the "freedom" side of the platform. While pleasant enough, Leo was the first guide who appeared to be only doing his job, and the bare minimum at that. While our previous guides eagerly participated in cultural exchanges and even sang with us, Leo escorted us to attractions, bought our tickets, then pointed to the door. After wandering around on our own, we would find him leaning against the taxi, smoking a cigarette, and talking on his cell phone.

Leo appeared to take some pride in telling us about his new cellphone. According to Leo, since the numbers six, eight, and nine are considered lucky in China, mobile phone numbers, license plates and apartments containing these three digits are more expensive. Meanwhile, the Chinese avoid the "deadly" number four, since the pronunciation of four (sì) sounds like the Chinese word for death (sǐ).

While many buildings in China lack a fourth floor, our ancient "culture hotel" in Suzhou had only two floors and our room was a safe number ten.

Tantamount to staying in a castle in Europe, a treehouse in the jungles of Central America, or that hotel where elephants wander through the lobby in Africa, our hotel in Suzhou wasn't just a hotel, it was a historical and cultural experience. The Pingjiang Lodge was so utterly charming I was willing to overlook numerous signs of age and a lack of modern comforts in order to experience life as a Chinese aristocrat.

Located in old Suzhou alongside a canal, the mansion was once owned by the Fang family during the Ming dynasty from 1368 to 1644 and was passed down through seven generations. The traditional Chinese courtyard manor has five halls, fifty-one rooms, eleven small gardens, and original quotes from the Little Red Book painted on the walls by Red Guards.

In the formal reception area, there was a brightly painted, porcelain set of Sanxing or "Three Stars." The three stars—Fu, Lu, and Shou—are the gods of prosperity, status, and longevity. Altars featuring these three gods are found in nearly every Chinese home and business, together with fortuitous offerings like oranges.

Fu is generally dressed as a scholar, holding a scroll or surrounded by children. Lu is dressed as an aristocratic Mandarin (with cool wing tips on his hat). Shou can be easily recognized as an old man with a huge forehead and a long white beard. He often holds a jade staff with a dragon's head and carries a peach or stands beside a deer or a crane. All three are symbols of longevity.

I had already purchased a set of Sanxing from our adoption agency but learned from Leo that they must be placed with Shou on the left, Lu in the middle, and Fu on the right (just as Chinese characters are traditionally written from right to left). Personally, my favorite is Fu, since his association with prosperity is based on personal gains from education and reproduction. In addition to my set of Sanxing, I placed a second statue of Fu next to my bed, for added luck in the parental prosperity department—at that point my nightstand was getting seriously cluttered.

All the antique Chinese furniture in our room had a butterfly motif. We slept in a beautifully carved cherry wood bed. The prehistoric Chinese "couch" looked more like a twin bed for toddlers. It had a decorative, carved wood rail bordering three sides of a thin, red, silk cushion on legs. Thankfully, two small throw pillows were provided for added "comfort." Quite possibly the first phone in China, a red triangle with a headset on top and a spinning dial, sat on a desk nearing the brink of collapse. The bathroom sink was a porcelain bowl painted with lily pads and koi fish atop an antique cabinet. The most interesting feature in the bathroom was the bathtub made out of wood.

Since it was raining when we arrived in Suzhou, Chris and I enjoyed a quiet, midday nap in our stateroom before exploring the grounds of our palatial estate. We wandered through the eleven courtyard gardens past small koi ponds, trickling rock fountains, white-sand Zen gardens, mini bamboo groves, and manicured bonsai trees. I tried my best to sign the guestbook using an ancient horse hair brush and an ink well, but I failed miserably.

We were living in the lap of luxury, at least by Ming dynasty standards.

While Hangzhou is famous for modern plant nurseries, Suzhou is the home of beautiful, classical Chinese gardens, several of which are world heritage sites. Suzhou used to boast over one hundred gardens. Sadly, only nine classical gardens remain in Suzhou, but they are over a thousand years old and provide a surreal glimpse into old-world China.

The intricately designed gardens were impressive, however, they proved difficult to see and fully appreciate in the pouring rain. The serenity of the gardens was further disrupted by the mass of tourists with giant umbrellas—sadly undeterred by the endless downpour.

Of all of Suzhou's elegant classical gardens none was more famous, grand, and award-winning than the Humble Administrator's Garden. Hailed as the mother of Chinese gardens, the nearly thirteen-acre garden was built in 1509 during the Ming dynasty by Wang Xianchen. He built the garden on top of the remains of the former residence of a Tang dynasty poet and an ancient temple from the Yuan dynasty. Being tired of life as a government official, he hoped to retire and live out the rest of his days relaxing in his garden. While it took sixteen years to design and build the garden, sadly he had only six years to enjoy the fruits of his labor before his son lost the estate due to gambling debts.

The garden was designed by a famous Chinese painter using concepts from art and poetry. From an aerial view, the elaborate garden was shaped like a dragon. A large lake sets the stage while small bamboo and pine forests, lush green hills, and large rock formations (as well as pavilions, bridges, and pagodas) create the backdrop. The former residence halls sit on stilts above the water connected by a network of covered bridges, rocky islands, and nature paths.

As we walked through a small bamboo forest next to a temple, I couldn't help but smile at seeing Chinese characters carved into the stalks of bamboo in the same way Americans carve initials of their sweethearts into tree trunks. Maybe we aren't so different after all?

In China, bamboo is a symbol for strength and is much admired for its resilience.

Take caution, however, while bamboo may be thought to be lucky, it's still a weed. Whether bamboo should be praised for its rapid growth is a matter of opinion. Chris' grandmother spent many years in Japan and traveling throughout Asia. Upon returning home to Virginia Beach, she planted bamboo in her garden, whereupon it took over the entire yard. According to Mee Maw Marian, "Anyone who plants bamboo gets what they deserve."

All classical Chinese gardens feature plants of happiness, namely plum and peach that represent the yang quality, as well as the king of flowers and personification of pure yang— the peony. The yin principle is most often represented by the chrysanthemum, a symbol of tranquility. The most popular aquatic flower is the lotus, due to its connection with Buddhism and purity and since it rises out of dark waters to bloom in the light. Hydrangeas, roses, narcissuses, camellias, hyacinths, orchids, and pomegranates are also widely used in classical Chinese gardens.

In addition, traditional Chinese gardens were designed with designated corners to be visited during each season. The summer section of a garden features broad leafed trees like ashes, oaks, and plantains that offer shade. The autumn sector highlights the intoxicating smell of mandarin trees and beautiful chrysanthemums. Winter landscapes are composed of frost-resistant plants and flowers and the noble pine tree. The spring sector boasts early roses, cherries, honeysuckle, almonds, violets, and narcissuses.

I thought of our small garden back home in Colorado. While our plum tree was thriving, our apple and peach trees had been struggling for years. The pots of river iris on the edge of our tiny pond were flourishing, but sadly the lotus flowers have been much less successful. I researched the lovely peony and was surprised to learn they grow at elevations up to seven thousand feet and actually require cold winters. Meanwhile, hardy chrysanthemums are one of the easiest perennials to grow. I don't have much of a green thumb, nor passion for gardening. During the Ming dynasty (1368-1644) it was written that "a flower is grown during a whole year but admired just ten days," (which pretty much sums up why I've never been a gardener, but I was determined to try to fill my garden with auspicious, Chinese flowers of happiness).

As testament to the completely opposite homes and lifestyles of my parents, they kept very different gardens (or rather didn't keep). At my father's estate, a Polish gardener/handyman tended a large lawn and beautiful rose garden. Every summer, before taking the bus to summer camp at Colorado Academy, I would pick a rose for the bus driver, Maggie. I would wrap the stem in a wet paper towel, before placing the precious bundle in a plastic sandwich bag. Then, I would present my cherished mother figure with my small but meaningful gift. My father never noticed that I was destroying his award-winning rose bushes.

Meanwhile, since next to nothing grows in New Mexico, my mother's garden consisted of artistically arranged rocks, Zen gardens of sand, rusted metal treasures, broken bits of pottery, a wide variety of wind chimes, and several Buddha statues (and lots and lots of cacti). In addition, my mother's yard had a dilapidated play structure, where my best friend and I used to play airline stewardess. We designed our own wind sock, created airline tickets, and jetted down the slide to fabulous vacations.

I will always love the smell of roses, but as a child, I preferred my mother's slightly lifeless but very creative and much-loved garden.

Suzhou's classic gardens reflect the ancient Chinese proverb that says In heaven there is paradise; on earth, Suzhou. The saying is indicative of the longstanding desire of the Chinese to create a version of heaven on earth by perfecting their natural environment. The symphonic combination of rocks, water, trees, and buildings in classical Chinese gardens demonstrates the Chinese appreciation of balance and harmony known as feng shui. *Feng* means "wind" or "breath of life" while *shui* is "water," an essential principal of life.

The concept of feng shui began during the Zhou dynasty (1027-777 BC) to determine auspicious grave sites and progressed to a method for finding appropriate dwelling sites. The main principle of feng shui stems from a Taoist belief in a single whole, involving heaven, earth, and man working in unison. Therefore, the key to a happy life is the coexistence of man and nature. The bonsai tree is a perfect example of this desire to cultivate and coexist with nature, but also perfect it.

The Chinese notion of yin and yang teaches that opposite but coexisting principles form the whole universe: dark and light, female and male, dead and alive. For a long time, the Chinese believed that the world was divided into four parts: Azure Dragon, Red Bird, Black Turtle and White Tiger. These four parts represented the four directions as well as the four seasons. By the third century BC, this idea led to the belief that the universe is composed of the five elements (wu xing) of wood, fire, earth, metal and water. All five elements have connections to the seasons, cardinal points, numbers, colors, internal organs, and more. Feng shui aims to achieve a balance of the opposing characteristics in the world around you, including the feminine yin and masculine yang, and the five elements and the energy force of qi. Feng Shui draws from astronomy, environmental science, and topography and combines elements of architecture, botany, ethics, and divination.

My desperation for a child had made me willing to try absolutely anything: expensive and invasive fertility treatments, a long and uncertain process to adopt, the infertility diet, meditation, massage, yoga and any and all fertility boosting practices, traditions and/or superstitions. I ate died-red sunflower seeds by the pound because to the Chinese they symbolize having lots of children (even though many Americans think red food dye causes attention deficit disorders).

If someone had told me eating raw eggs with seaweed, turning around three times with your eyes closed and then standing on your head in a southeast direction would get you pregnant, I would have happily tried it—again and again and again.

One of my first efforts to reach my goal to have a child was to fully embrace the art of feng shui and thus harmonize my environment in all ways that related to fertility.

Since Chris and I were both born during the Year of the Ox, our birth element is water. Therefore, I completely redecorated our home with shades of blue and added numerous water features: pictures of water, tabletop fountains, and mirrors. I positioned our bed in a northwest direction (north toward heaven and west toward the future), cleared an energy path to the front door, and removed "fire" objects from the west sector associated with children. I hung a crystal over the entrance to the master bathroom to prevent our luck from washing down the many drains. Plus, I placed a pair of lucky elephants at the door to our bedroom, symbols of double fish for marital bliss all over the house, and a single piece of hollow bamboo in the north sector of our bedroom.

And for the finishing touch, I put a dragon statue on my husband's nightstand to add extra baby-generating oomph to our lovemaking.

While classical Chinese gardens were designed to accommodate air and light quality, noise levels, angles of the sun, the five elements of Taoism, the Chinese zodiac, and the principles of feng shui, all of that pales in comparison to the balancing act mandated by fertility treatments. In my opinion, the precise timing, detailed medications, complicated science, and fragile susceptibility of fertility treatments make rocket science (and classical Chinese gardening) look easy.

Each of my IVF cycles started with two to three weeks of taking birth control pills, which always seemed very counterintuitive to me. Then around day twenty-one, came the down phase, when I took Lupron to suppress hormone production and ovarian function (and got headaches, night sweats, and serious mood swings). Next, came the baseline ultrasound and blood test to check my estradiol value. If my level was normal, I was then cleared for the stimulation phase. For ten to twelve days, I became a human pin cushion as Chris injected me with gonadotropin meds to stimulate my ovaries to mass-produce eggs, then another round of injections to avoid premature release of the eggs. The doctors had to strictly monitor the thickness of my uterine lining and number of developing follicles.

In addition to looking like a walking punching bag, my breasts grew tender and my stomach became bloated. Then thirty-seven hours before egg retrieval, I was given a trigger shot of the human pregnancy hormone (human chorionic gonadotropin) to mature my eggs and stimulate ovulation. Finally, my eggs were retrieved via a needle guided by ultrasound. Chris offered up his swimmers, then via the ICSI process (Intracytoplasmic Sperm Injection, a specialized add-on to in vitro fertilization to one-up Mother Nature) the best and brightest sperm were injected directly into my eggs. The fertilized eggs were then incubated and grown. Finally, after three to five days, the highest quality embryos were transferred to my womb (and any remaining embryos were put on ice).

All of this painstakingly precise effort, with high physical, emotional, and financial demands, resulted in a one out of three chance of actually getting pregnant.

So the next time someone asks you what ancient Chinese classical gardens, modern fertility treatments, and rocket science have in common, you can respond:

They are *astronomically* complicated.

The Chinese have a long tradition of honoring flowers and plants. During the Double Ninth (Chongyang) Festival, celebrated on the ninth day of the ninth lunar month, Chinese people gather to admire blooming chrysanthemums, take hikes and picnics in the mountains, and visit gravesites to prepare the spirits for winter. On this day, the Chinese repeat the traditions of Qing Ming, but this time they blanket the graves in bright yellow chrysanthemums, the flower of the autumn moon.

As with all Chinese festivals, there is a legend attached to the Day of the Double Sun, representing the end of autumn. During the Eastern Han dynasty, the God of Plague, who lived in the Nu River, caused disease in the surrounding villages. The parents of a young scholar named Heng Jing (Huan Jing) died because of the devil's black magic. Heng Jing went through great lengths to find an immortal or wise monk to teach him swordsmanship, so he could vanquish the devil.

On the ninth day of the ninth lunar month, the villagers climbed over a mountain, to the river, prepared with leaves of dogwood and cups of chrysanthemum wine. When the God of Plague appeared, he was distracted by the fragrance. Whereupon, Heng Jing attacked with his demon-slaying Green Dragon Sword, defeated the devil and ended the plague. (In a second, rather unimaginative version, Huan Jing simply took the villagers on a picnic in the mountains, to escape from harm).

Drinking chrysanthemum wine is an important part of the festival, since the flowers are thought to be an antitoxin that can drive away evil. The festival is also celebrated with chongyang cake, a steamed cake with layers of nuts and jujube (Chinese red dates). Since the word *gao* means both cake and high in Chinese, many people choose to climb tall mountains to eat cake and drink chrysanthemum wine in order to cure disease, prevent disaster, and achieve *higher* personal awareness and achievement.

Staying true to my future daughter's Chinese roots while being raised in the United States would surely come with many challenges. Thankfully, with five different Asian markets in the Denver area, tracking down a chongyang cake and chrysanthemum wine to celebrate the Double Ninth Festival wouldn't be too difficult (and there is always the wonderous Internet). When it comes to climbing mountains to gain personal awareness, the State of Colorado wrote the book. And the bright yellow glow of aspen trees in the fall is a fitting substitute for chrysanthemums (in the likely case I fail to grow them).

Since the number nine means long or everlasting in Chinese, it represents longevity, and therefore the Double Ninth Festival is also designated as Senior's Day. Families accompany their elders to outdoor settings and wish them health and happiness on this joyous day.

In China, my name is associated with drinking flower wine, eating cake, taking a hike, and celebrating seniors, as well as, being the favorite number of the emperors and associated with the concepts of longevity and completeness. Not too shabby!

My memories of Suzhou are its picturesque canals, living like a Chinese millionaire in an authentic Ming dynasty mansion, eating lots of dumplings, and rain—lots and lots of rain.

There's an American saying that April showers bring May flowers (and a Colorado saying that April showers bring May blizzards), and while visiting Suzhou in April it rained every day. Our umbrellas became our constant companions; however, the travel umbrellas we packed in case of rain were not holding up well in actual rain. But the Chinese have a saying, You wouldn't want to be a *luò tāng jī,* or a "drop soup chicken," who gets caught in the rain (and looks like a soaking wet chick or a drowned rat).

The rain was no longer misty and magical, it was cold, dark, and extremely vexing. Our shoes were soaked, our clothes were wet, our daypacks were soggy, and our noses were dripping. I bought several bars of Bee & Flower soap, with scents like jasmine and ginseng, and placed them throughout my backpack to freshen my damp clothing. Having grown up in the Southwest, in a land rumored to have 365 days of sunshine and the world's most magnificent sunrises and sunsets, I was ill prepared for constant rain and was starting to go insane—but at least it wasn't windy!

Most tourists who visit Suzhou come for its famed classical gardens. While the gardens of Suzhou were certainly lovely, they weren't exactly peaceful. In their defense, any garden would fall short of serenity while under siege by visitors toting video cameras, giant handbags, and noisy cell phones. Even in the pouring rain, the Humble Administrator's Garden was full to bursting, making it impossible to cross the lovely Small Flying Rainbow Bridge and difficult to find any sense of beauty and tranquility. (And there's nothing like cold water dripping down your back to dampen your outfit, mood and level of appreciation.) So we moved on to a private boat tour of the Grand Canal, which turned out to be much more relaxing and enjoyable, even though it was still raining.

Considered to be the oldest and longest man-made canal in the world, the 1,115-mile Grand Canal flows from Beijing to Hangzhou and links five rivers, including the Yangtze and the Yellow River, and fifteen major cities. With a history of over twenty-five-hundred years, the canal was begun in 468 BC and went through three major phases of renovation and expansion during the Spring and Autumn period (770 BC-476 BC), the Sui dynasty (581-618), and the Yuan dynasty (1271-1368).

With the goal of linking northern and southern China, the Mongolian emperors during the Yuan dynasty ordered more than four million slaves to finish the Grand Canal, most of whom died of disease and exhaustion after ten years of hard labor. Upon completion of the Grand Canal, foreign trade flourished, technology advanced, and China became extremely prosperous. So, the hostile Mongolian takeover and reign of Khublai Khan wasn't all bad (as long as you weren't a soldier, slave, or generally unlucky commoner).

Emperor Sui Yangdi is said to have celebrated the completion of the canal by touring it on a flotilla of dragon boats pulled by the empire's most beautiful women. While the grand affair may have been a bit outlandish and tawdry (and some claim the emperor's extravagance brought down the Sui dynasty), there was due cause for revelry, as the Grand Canal belt continues to be one of the richest agricultural areas in China. Suzhou has greatly prospered due to the Grand Canal, and the Jiangsu province has been dubbed the land of fish and rice.

Marco Polo, it seems, had a bit of a crush on China; in addition to Hangzhou, he also had a love of Suzhou and called it the Venice of the East. As our tour boat driver left the Grand Canal and began to maneuver through the ancient, narrow waterways that dissect old Suzhou, it became clear why Suzhou gained its nickname, for it truly began to look like the famous Italian city of canals.

While the canals of Venice and Suzhou look strikingly similar, everything else about the landscape was distinctively Chinese. We floated past ancient temples and under moon-shaped bridges. We passed alongside a waterfront boardwalk park filled with blooming trees, sitting pavilions, and enormous rock sculptures and lined with ornate wrought-iron street lights decorated with red lanterns. We passed numerous tiny bamboo rafts and large dragon boats (but no long, thin gondolas with Italians in striped shirts and flat straw hats).

Just like in Venice, the ancient homes that rose from the edge of the canals appeared as though they could crumble and sink into the water at any moment. The bases of the white homes bordering the canals were darkly stained by water, algae, and time; plants creeped through large cracks in the foundations and window boxes and balconies sagged dangerously close to the water's surface. There was a group of homes completely covered in vines, and their windows appeared to be sealed shut. Several homes, precariously perched atop brick retaining walls, were missing a frightening number of bricks. The bottom tiers of a stairway leading down to the water looked like they were melting. Death-defying but beautiful covered wooden walkways crossed over the canals, linking tiny alleys and almost clipped the top of our boat. Locals on top of small, arched bridges huddled under umbrellas and took pictures of us as we passed underneath, and we took photographs of them.

According to the boatman, there were more than one thousand bridges in Suzhou. Due to the number of canals, area water towns still held daily boat markets where goods were sold directly from the decks of tiny rafts and large fishing boats. In old-town Suzhou, many of the homes had Internet and cable but no running water. Some of the homes had no showers or toilets and residents still used a bed pan.

As someone with a small bladder that can't make it through a night without several trips to the toilet, I had to seriously question the priorities of the residents of old Suzhou. For access to hot showers and not having to use a bed pan under any circumstances, let alone in the middle of the night, I would happily sacrifice Facebook and HBO. However, Chris would sooner use a bedpan than give up *Game of Thrones*.

11

SILKEN LEGENDS
AND DUMPLING DREAMS

In addition to classical gardens and flowing canals, Suzhou is also known as the Pink City and Hometown of Silk, which was once the most coveted textile on Earth. Great empires sent merchants across oceans and deserts to travel East along the Silk Road in pursuit of the prized cloth, and they paid for it by weight like gold.

We visited the state-owned, No. 1 Silk Factory founded in 1926, where workers continued to unravel silkworm cocoons by hand, as has been done for thousands of years. As part of a tour, we were able to hold live silkworms, touch a variety of cocoons, and help stretch newly woven raw silk.

Leo told us that up until 1949 (when China became a Communist country), very few men living in Suzhou worked. Silk was the main industry in Suzhou and only women were hired for their higher level of patience (much like with the tea industry). At that time, roughly eight out of ten women in Suzhou worked in the silk industry. Meanwhile, the men simply spent their days at teahouses and going to shows.

Today, billions of silkworms must be cultivated every year to support China's silk industry. Female moths lay 350 to 400 tiny eggs, then promptly die. The eggs are incubated for ten days, then upon hatching, the worms begin to feast on mulberry leaves. After around six weeks of constantly eating, the worms quadruple in size (to roughly three inches) and begin to spin cocoons.

While constructing its cocoon, the silkworm will twist in a figure eight motion roughly three hundred thousand times to produce several thousand feet of filament in a single strand. Sadly, the process of hatching destroys the cocoon, therefore to harvest the silk, cocoons are boiled in water, which loosens the filament but kills the pupae. Then, machines spin the silk filament into skeins, with a cocoon attached to each spindle. The filament of each cocoon must remain unbroken.

A single pound of silk requires the lives of some twenty-five hundred silkworms. Often the dead silkworms are seasoned, boiled or fried, and eaten—so at least no part of the ill-fated silkworm is wasted.

China continues to lead the world in silk production, producing roughly fifty-eight thousand tons each year or about three-quarters of the world's supply of raw silk. Nearly 80 percent of the world's bridal gowns come from Suzhou and are available at wholesale prices from more than a thousand wedding stores in the city. As a hopeful future mother, I was more in the market for silken baby blankets, adorable onesies, and tiny booties (of which I already had plenty secretly stashed in the guest bedroom closet).

In the silk factory gift shop, I found the perfect tiger hat with pop-up ears. In addition to the Five Deadly Animals, tigers are believed to protect and watch over infants, and are as popular in China as Pooh Bear and Mickey Mouse are in the USA. Chinese grandmothers have been known to sew gold, silver, and jade charms onto infant tiger hats to protect their grandchildren. The hat I bought was adorable. (I only wished it came with a Chinese grandmother).

I was tempted to buy a silk scarf, since I'd developed a cold thanks to the constant rain in Suzhou, not to mention our historic but drafty accommodations. But I discovered that my conscience prefers wool, since sheep merely suffer a haircut.

While visiting the No. 1 Silk Factory, I read The Story of Silk on a plaque below a woman's portrait labeled the Goddess of Silkworms and the whimsical tale behind the chance discovery of silk gave me much to contemplate.

According to legend, the unexpectedly fortuitous idea of harvesting thread from silkworms was discovered by Xi Ling Shi, the Empress Leizu, wife of the Yellow Emperor, around 2,700 BC. It's said that she discovered the ancient secret when a silkworm cocoon fell into her cup of tea. Softened in the hot liquid, the cocoon began to unravel. As she pulled the cocoon out of her tea, the empress inadvertently discovered silk thread.

This revelation led to the planting of groves of mulberry trees, the fabrication of looms, and the establishment of a silk industry—all powered by the women of China. And for discovering the secret of the silkworm cocoon, Xi Ling Shi was given the title Seine-Than, or Goddess of Silkworms.

As I read, I found myself thinking, who does this? Who reacts to a worm falling into their cup of tea, by studying the wet cocoon, rather than immediately tossing it out and ordering a cup of coffee instead?

I'm not sure whether there is any truth to this story or not, but there's something about it that resonates with me. The empress didn't freak out about a bug landing in her tea, instead she calmly observed the small creature. She realized the potential within the little cocoon and her vision led to the creation of a world-dominating, silk industry. It's a wonderful example of seeing the potential for a life lesson and being open to a new journey, even when life takes a detour.

Xi Ling Shi's story speaks to me because I want to be that person. I want to have a silver-lining (or a silken-thread) mindset. I want to embrace that kind of spontaneous journey in my own life.

When dealing with infertility, it's easy to focus on a singular path, putting all your hopes upon the latest procedure, newest doctor, or trending fertility-boosting superstition. Then, when your efforts fail, you blindly follow the next potential solution until that effort crashes and burns and in desperation you latch onto yet another possible miracle—and the vicious cycle continues. Then, as doors continually slam in your face, you become blind to open windows.

Perhaps navigating through the trials of life with eyes wide open to unexpected possibilities is a healthier, happier option. According to J.R.R. Tolkien (and a variety of Phish and Jeep bumper stickers), "not all who wander are lost." In my humble opinion, tunnel vision seems more likely to lead you into a head-on encounter with a train.

As renowned as China is for silk, dumplings are a tradition that may be lesser known internationally but are woven just as solidly into the fabric of the culture.

A word of caution, don't bite into a Chinese dumpling; the boiling hot juice will squirt you in the face, burn your lips, and leave behind grease on your clothes. Better to nibble a small hole in one end and suck out the juice before devouring the dumpling whole. This is the valuable lesson we learned while dining at the Yang Yang Dumpling Restaurant. It was our last night in Suzhou, and we ventured out in the rain to obtain dinner, on our own. Thankfully our Lonely Planet guidebook steered us to the dumpling restaurant, which the locals seemed to approve of as it was completely full, and we were the only tourists. The restaurant offered a huge menu (with English translations) and a very festive atmosphere, plus it was open until 3:00 a.m.

While the menu was absolutely enormous (with roughly a hundred options from which to choose), we only counted five types of dumplings, so we're not exactly sure why it was called a dumpling restaurant. We greatly enjoyed a feast of sweet and sour chicken, pork and vegetable dumplings, spicy garlic fried green beans (which we were thrilled to enjoy a second time, though not as spicy as in Xi'an), fried rice, and egg rolls. The food was incredible, and we noticed the locals ordered the same dishes as us, so we were feeling pretty good about ourselves.

China has been perfecting the art of dumpling making since the Song dynasty (960-1127). Jiaozi, or Chinese dumplings, typically consist of a ground meat and/or vegetable filling wrapped in a thin piece of dough. Dumplings are eaten with a soy-sauce-based dip that may include sesame oil, vinegar, rice wine, hot sauce, garlic, and ginger. Jiaozi may be round or crescent-shaped, boiled or pan-fried, sweet or savory.

Jiaozi are one of the most important and traditional dishes in China. It is said there are twenty-six different kinds of jiaozi, since there are twenty-six different festivals throughout the year where eating a specific dumpling is part of the celebration. From food-based festivals including the Cold Food and Lychee and Dog Meat festivals (yep, dog meat) to the Dragon Boat, Torch and Kite festivals, and the Nine Emperor Gods and Monkey King festivals dumplings play a major role.

The most important annual festival is the Chinese New Year, where Chinese families cast out the old and welcome in the new, while consuming a large quantity of dumplings. Traditionally known as the Spring Festival, the fifteen-day celebration begins on the first new moon and continues until the first full moon (sometime between January 19 and February 23).

Festivities begin with the Kitchen God ritual (more on him later), followed by settling debts (based on the Chinese proverb If a little money is not spent, great money will not be realized) and cleaning house for a fresh start (always finishing by New Year's Eve to avoid sweeping away any New Year's luck). Next, the Chinese decorate with "lucky paper" wall hangings and couplets with wishes for good fortune, buy a new (most likely red) party outfit, and feast with loved ones.

Adults give children "lucky money" in ornate, red envelopes. Good luck is thought to follow both those who give and those who receive.

Signifying unity and harmony, the New Year's Eve dinner is considered the most important family ritual of the year. It is believed that if a family doesn't share a New Year's Eve dinner together, the family's love will grow cold.

A menu including eight courses is considered auspicious since in Chinese the word for eight sounds like to grow. Meats like chicken and fish are served *yu* or whole, which sounds like the word for abundance. Meat dishes include the head and tail, so as not to be broken, which is unlucky. Long-grain rice, noodles, and string beans are often served to ensure a long life.

The featured dessert is a gelatinous rice cake, decorated with yams, dates, and nuts. The cake is called *nian gao*, or "year cake" and represents reaching for a better life since *gao* sounds like the word for high. This traditional cake, while similar to a Christmas fruitcake, is much more revered (and is never re-gifted to an unpopular Aunt, passed around at office white elephant parties, or used by children to play hot potato).

Chinese families begin eating special New Year's yuanbao dumplings just after midnight on the New Year. Red candles illuminate the house so bad luck can't creep inside and ancestral spirits are fed at the family altar. Lucky family members bite into dumplings and discover a fortune. Popular fortunes include one of eight symbolic items: *peanuts* for a long life, *candy* for a sweet life, *dimes* for prosperity, *red dates* for luck, *dried logan fruit* for achievement, *rice cake* for promotion, *oranges* for positive outcomes, and *walnuts* for peace. While boiling, it's imperative that the dumplings not break, or the family's wealth and luck could fall out.

Since whole families often participate in making the yuanbao, the dumplings have come to represent unity, harmony, and balance.

I must confess, I'm a terrible cook and pretty much subsist on hummus. (If it weren't for Amy's frozen entrees, I'd be near starving.) Chris claims I can't even boil water (and he's right, I left a pot of water to boil for so long it burned a hole through the bottom of the pot, and I had to discard the evidence).

However, I had high hopes that I could master the art of making Chinese dumplings so that one day I could make yuanbao every year with my husband and children. After all, I have fond memories of being a teenager making "assembly-line" eggrolls with my family. My younger half sisters stuffed, I wrapped, and my mom fried. It was quiet the production.

It's fascinating how the traditions of your childhood linger long into your adult years, and even shape the kinds of memories you long to create with your own children. My mother, whose great-grandparents emigrated from Sweden, tried her best to keep us connected to our Scandinavian roots while living in New Mexico. Therefore, most years we would celebrate St. Lucia Day on December 13.

Lucia can be traced to the martyr St. Lucia of Italy (which works out well since my half sisters are part Italian), but modern Swedes celebrate her as the bearer of light during cold, dark Scandinavian winters. Legend tells of a young woman wearing a white dress and crown of candles who braved the snow to bring food to the people.

As the oldest daughter, I got to be St. Lucia. I rose early, dressed in a long white nightgown with a red sash and a crown, then served breakfast to my family. Each year, my mother and I would collect pine branches from the yard to fashion a crown of light (we tried candles but quickly went electric). The night before, we would make biscuits and cinnamon rolls, which my little sisters called stickies, or sometimes go to the European bakery for lussekatter, sweet saffron buns that look like curled-up cats with raisin eyes. My sisters would sneak out of bed to be my handmaidens or Lucy girls, but sadly we didn't have any star boys with tall, white, conical hats and star wands. We would sing the St. Lucia Song and eat breakfast together.

Oddly enough, I have become closer to my Swedish roots after marrying my husband, simply because he speaks Swedish. He used to meet with Swedish exchange students at CU-Boulder for conversation, and thereby we have established a large group of Swedish friends, traveled to Sweden together to attend a wedding, and regularly attend the local mid-Summer festival in Estes Park.

As Chris and I left the dumpling restaurant and headed back to our room in our historical manor, it dawned on me that if I could master the art of making Chinese dumplings, my dreams for my future family would include American, Chinese, Hispanic, German, French and Scandinavian traditions.

Welcome to the melting pot, baby girl!

Before leaving Suzhou, we took one last trip to the local convenience store, in pursuit of the standard dessert, toxic alcohol, and random souvenir purchases. We were not disappointed.

We found a large white bottle of nose-hair-singeing alcohol with a lovely landscape of Southern China painted in bright blue. I also came across the Chinese version of the friendship necklace found at cheap jewelry stores in the States. The Best Friends pendant consists of a metal heart charm broken into two equal halves and worn by two best friends. The significantly lovelier and more upscale, Chinese convenience store version consisted of two equal pieces of white stone carved with delicate flowers and Chinese characters. I redesigned the broken heart charm into earrings but hoped to one day share the best friends token with my daughter.

Best of all we discovered the ancient art of fortune sticks. They are thin pieces of bamboo with red tips and bizarre fortunes written in rudimentary English on one side and Chinese characters on the other side. Chris and I were delighted by the array of memorable fortunes:

"You will have a bad dream, but no harm will follow."

"Being vain will cause you pain."

"Your love 'interets' are wrong and soon will be right."

But my favorites were "Changes every seven 'year' will occur to you" and "A man and woman will shortly annoy you."

We bought a package of the bamboo sticks to take home with us. I had no doubt that rereading the humorous fortunes would be a source of never-ending delight. But I think that what I love best about the bamboo fortune sticks is the way they smell. One whiff and I am transported back to Suzhou, past the gardens, and beyond the canals, until I can imagine myself standing in the middle of a bamboo forest deep in the heart of China.

12

CROSSING BRIDGES
AND LEAPING WATERFALLS

If Suzhou is known as the Venice of the East, then the nearby water town of Tongli is the Italian city's miniature, Chinese doppelgänger.

On our way to our final destination of Shanghai, we spent several pleasant hours in the ancient water town where nearly every building bordered a canal.

The town was originally named Futu or "rich land," but the name was thought to be vulgar and therefore was changed to Tongli, which means "copper." Built during the Song dynasty (960-1279), Tongli is surrounded by five lakes and is divided into seven islands by fifteen canals, which inspired the building of forty-nine picturesque bridges.

Many local traditions revolve around the bridges of Tongli. It is customary for locals to walk across The Three Bridges during times of celebration, such as weddings, births and traditional festivals. The Taiping Bridge, or Peace and Tranquility Bridge, is said to bring good health. The arched Jili Bridge or Luck Bridge, inscribed with couplets heralding the beautiful view, is thought to increase prosperity. The Changqing Bridge or Lasting Celebration Bridge affords an evergreen life for the coming year. The trio of bridges crossed three rivers at their confluence and formed a natural ring road.

As I walked across the symbolic bridges, I had a vision of one day standing on the tallest bridge, holding my infant daughter high above my head, into a ray of light, just like the baboon Rafiki in the movie *Lion King* when he presented Simba atop Pride Rock.

Chris and I held hands as we crossed over the most magical bridge in town, Fuguan Bridge. This bridge features a stone carving called the Fish Fossil in the Peach Blossom Wave. The carving depicts the legend of a humble fish that swam against the current of a peach blossom–covered river in hopes of becoming an immortal dragon by jumping over the Dragon Gate. However, as the fish sprang from the water, it was distracted by a beautiful girl standing on the bridge; therefore, its head was above the gate and became a dragon head while its body was below the gate and remained as a fish.

In Chinese mythology, fish and dragons share a deep bond, and the dragon is head of the fish clan. According to folklore, if a carp could leap the waterfall along the Yellow River at Dragon Gate, it would transform into a dragon. Many ancient Chinese believed that fish competed in an annual competition to leap the Longmen Falls and become dragons. This story came to symbolize success in the arduous civil service exams and images of fish leaping over waterfalls are still popular in China.

The story of the Chinese carp sounds a lot like the North American salmon's annual upstream battle against the forces of nature. I have always been inspired by the salmon's fierce determination to survive swimming against the current, past multiple predators, to lay their eggs and continue their species. If carp can leap waterfalls to become dragons and salmon can swim upstream to lay their eggs, maybe there was hope that I could become a mother.

It was stories like these that fostered my resolve to never give up.

Many of the scenic, pedestrian-only streets in Tongli are lined with canals on both sides, and down the center are shops, teahouses, and open-air restaurants with patios full of multicolored umbrellas. Vendors on boats pulled up to the banks of the canals and attempted to sell goods directly off their crafts. Plus, the streets were stuffed with makeshift stalls, small tents and rows of tables filled with artwork, clothing, and souvenirs. In the end, it was a complete quagmire through which locals and tourists alike could barely navigate.

Narrow pathways wound their way throughout Tongli between the streets and canals. Cangchang Lane had a riverbank at each end and was so narrow that only one person could walk along it at a time, earning it the nickname One Person Lane.

The canals were completely clogged with small flat boats, while their banks were lined with yards upon yards of clothesline. As we walked, we passed several women with large woven baskets washing clothes in the canals. According to Leo, the Chinese preferred drying their clothes in "fresh" air as opposed to using machine dryers. The clotheslines filled with random, colorful clothing throughout China were known as national flags.

As we wandered the charming streets of Tongli, I asked Leo about a strange wooden apparatus sitting outside a small restaurant alongside a mini fridge filled with soda. The antique device had two circular grey stones on top, a long crank sticking out the side, and a piece of cheese cloth hanging over the front. A pile of yellow beans sat in the middle of the stone on top and a river of foamy, white goop oozed out from underneath the bottom stone. He informed us that the bizarre and rather unsanitary-looking device was for making tofu.

I grew up eating tofu (before it was a health trend). I remember my mother making tofu pumpkin pie at Thanksgiving, eating tofu pups instead of hot dogs and getting Tofutti ice cream at the health food store. During elementary school, I often had sleepovers at the home of a friend whose family ran an indoor soy bean farm (both her parents had long dreadlocks which they tied up with scarves). But I hadn't eaten tofu in years, not since I began struggling to get pregnant. Soy consumption by women has been controversial due to its large content of isoflavones, a compound that acts like estrogen in the body. Some studies claim soy disrupts hormone balances while other studies tout benefits for women trying to conceive. I had erred on the side of caution and carefully monitored my soy consumption. Now, seeing tofu being made in this rustic fashion made me rethink my love of the gelatinous food. As for Chris, I'd never been able to get him to try the stuff. I was pretty sure that, now, I never would.

Our home back in Colorado was already a jumbled mess of folk art from travels in Europe and Central America, my Scandinavian ancestry, and my sentimental obsession with Mexican handicrafts.

We didn't need one more thing.

Then we visited a jade factory and a cloisonné workshop, both unscheduled stops on our tour itinerary, which we found to be fascinating insights into the incredible artistry of China—and the perfect place to indulge my penchant for Asian art.

In China, jade is considered a celestial jewel that bridges heaven and earth. It had been a symbol of status, spirituality, and health for more than nine thousand years and was rumored to possess supernatural powers. It was said that wearing jade in the shape of a butterfly could attract love, and jade was given as a gift to formalize engagements. I purchased a pale green, jade, butterfly pendant in hopes of attracting a baby to love and planned to one day give the pendant to my child to celebrate our union.

"You should wear jade on your left, so it is close to your heart," the jeweler told us. "Chinese children wear a jade pendant of their Chinese zodiac animal as their protector, so at age twelve, after they've been through the full zodiac calendar, they aren't taken back by the gods."

I thought of my babies that had been "taken back by the gods" before they even had a chance to receive a zodiac animal protector. I wondered what the zodiac symbol of my future Chinese daughter would be or if that information would be known. I was tempted to buy bracelets of all twelve zodiac animals, just to be on the safe side.

Instead, we purchased a dark green jade happiness ball, which is a ball with smaller balls inside. The outer ball is decoratively carved with a dragon and a phoenix. There are window-like holes so that one can see the next ball inside. Then there are holes in that ball to see the smaller ball within that ball. It's like an ornate, round, three-dimensional puzzle. Each of the three balls represent one generation of a family and all the balls are entwined together in one piece. Happiness balls take two weeks to carve and cost a small fortune. According to a Chinese proverb, Gold has a price; jade is priceless.

At a cloisonné factory, we added more family-themed treasures to our international art collection. Cloisonné, so exquisite and vibrant, was once reserved only for the royal family. The art of cloisonné involved numerous challenging and time-consuming steps. First, artists made a copper vessel (a vase, medallion, or plate), then covered it with intricate, curved, copper wire designs. Next, they added colored enamel sand to create an image. Then they sent the vessels through eight rounds of firing at one thousand degrees, adding more sand after each trip to the oven, since the sand shrinks in the heat. Lastly, the works of art were polished and often gold plated.

After witnessing the multiple painstaking steps to crafting cloisonné, I had a much truer appreciation for the art form and higher tolerance for the accompanying price tag. We wandered around the gift shop for the better part of an hour before Chris finally chose a traditional happy marriage vase with a phoenix and dragon. The pair represents the perfect match, as yin is to yang, heaven is to earth, moon is to sun, and woman is to man. I chose small, moon-shaped, Buddha-like figures of a Chinese boy and girl.

The butterfly pendant, happiness ball, marriage vase, and twin children figurines were added to the growing number of souvenirs we purchased while in China that represent happy marriage, family, and love. Without realizing it, I was drawn to these items; purchasing symbols of family warmed my heart, gave me comfort, and surrounded me with little visuals of hope. There's nothing like longing for a baby to make you believe in the power of visualization. I hoped that surrounding myself with symbols of what I craved would ultimately bring that desire to fruition.

13

TALES OF THE KITCHEN GOD

Every autumn, the Chinese go completely mental over little, furry crustaceans!

Hairy crab, also known as the Chinese mitten crab, is one of the most prized delicacies in southeastern Chinese cuisine. The crabs are only in season two months out of the year, from roughly late September to mid-November, making the crustaceans extremely coveted. Each year, Leo and his family race to Tongli during the height of the hairy crab season to snatch up the biggest and best crabs.

The burrowing crab is native to the rivers of eastern Asia. Roughly the size of a human palm, the crab has a dark green back and distinctive brown fur on its golden mitten-like claws. In autumn, the hairy crab reaches maturity and migrates from its freshwater habitat to the ocean—leading to a massive and lucrative hunt by local gourmands and the culinary industry.

Hairy crabs are beloved by the Chinese for their sweet meat and buttery roe (eggs). The traditional recipe for hairy crabs is a simple one: steam and eat with a rice vinegar and ginger sauce.

According to Leo, a crab's price is based on its size and location (the body of water where each crab originates has its own reputation). The most coveted and therefore expensive crabs are females from the Yangcheng Lake in Jiangsu Province. The skyrocketing value of the crustaceans has led to fake crabs, known as bath crabs, being passed off as Yangcheng Lake crabs (because seriously, how would anyone know the difference?).

During the height of the hairy crab frenzy, the crustaceans can be found at every market and in every restaurant and are the most sought-after Mid-Autumn Festival gift. They were even sold in vending machines at subway stations in Nanjing. They were sold live (but in a deep freeze) for around twenty yuan (three dollars), along with the appropriate accoutrements of vinegar and two bags of ginger tea.

Having been raised in a high desert, mountainous climate, the first time I visited Chris' family in St. Mary' County, Maryland, I felt like I was in a foreign country; I had no experience with oyster festivals and clambakes. The Maryland Blue Crab is a truly gorgeous specimen with an iridescent green body and bright blue arms and legs; plus, the females have red "nail polish" on the tips of their claws. I always have fun going crabbin'. We lure the crabs with rubbery turkey leftovers on a string and then catch them in a large net. I shriek and holler to the great amusement of the local fishing community. However, while I enjoy catching crabs and watching kids chase each other around with crab claws, I'll be damned if I ever eat crabs or any seafood for that matter.

I may have grown up in the Rocky Mountains, but I have deep southern roots, no matter how tangled. I was born in Houston, Texas, to a father from Louisiana, who seemed to think eating seafood defined our family. Once, when I was seven, my father insisted that I eat a raw oyster. I had no idea whether to bite it or swallow it whole (and was too scared to ask for guidance). Long story short, a staff member of the Cherry Creek Country Club had to give me the Heimlich maneuver (and I was thoroughly reprimanded for causing a scene). Then, when I was eleven, my father took me to the World's Fair in New Orleans. After a day of riding roller coasters, he made me eat seafood gumbo and I vomited all over a five-star restaurant in the French Quarter (and was again reprimanded for my shockingly indelicate behavior).

Throughout my childhood, I remember being brought to tears by my father's claims that I was adopted and wasn't a true Southerner because I didn't like seafood. To this day, I can't stand seafood (but love pecan pie, black-eyed peas and grits!).

Like the perpetually doomed silkworm, the unfortunate hairy crab is an unwilling yet essential participant in China's fascinating culture. However, this one Chinese tradition would likely not be a part of our daughter's upbringing, since we wouldn't be having hairy crabs in Colorado, or in my case, ever. However, I looked forward to taking my daughter crabbin' when we'd visit her grandparents in Maryland.

❀

Teahouses are to China, what outdoor cafés are to France, and pubs are to Great Britain (and microbreweries are to Colorado).

There was a plethora of charming, water-front, restaurants to choose from in Tongli. We chose to have lunch at the Nanyuan Teahouse, which was part restaurant and part museum and looked like it could have been part of the set for the movie *Crouching Tiger, Hidden Dragon*. The large, two-story establishment built during the Qing dynasty was said to be the first teahouse in the Jiangnan region. It looked like a pavilion floating between two canals.

According to Leo, during the early morning hours, the restaurant is filled with local seniors eating breakfast, drinking tea, and sharing the news and gossip of the day. In addition, local fishermen frequent the location, giving it the nickname fisherman's pier.

The back wall of the restaurant was stacked to the ceiling with traditional Chinese rice buckets, bamboo pails that looked very much like the buckets found inside of Scandinavian saunas and at upscale day spas. Traditionally, small single-compartment boxes with lids and handles were used to carry lunch portions of rice, while larger boxes with no lids transported rice from the fields. From the looks of the stacks of rice buckets, the restaurant supplied numerous locals with lunches to go.

I searched antique stores all over China in hopes of finding an authentic, multi-compartment lunch box with the idea to use it as a unique jewelry box. I had specifically hoped to find boxes with auspicious symbols for family and children. To my great disappointment, the boxes I found were either too large, falling apart, or very expensive (or all three). Oh well, I don't own that much jewelry anyway. (Plus, nothing could beat the red, metal Nancy Drew lunch box, complete with a spooky lighthouse on a cliff, I had in grade school. It was totally rad.)

In the back of the restaurant was also an old-world kitchen with an ancient kiln for boiling drinking water over a wood fire. In the past, it was cheaper and easier for locals to buy the day's supply of drinking water from the teahouse than to burn wood and boil their own. The kiln hadn't been used in years but was kept clean and stocked to show visitors a glimpse of forgotten China.

The establishment also had a display of beautiful antique teapots and a traditional teahouse bar filled with several rows of tins and porcelain jars of tea. There was a stage for regional Kunqu opera performances, private rooms partitioned with bamboo and silk screens, and not one but two shrines to the Kitchen God.

While the Elf on the Shelf magically appears in many American homes with children to elicit good behavior during the winter holiday season, the Chinese believe in the Kitchen God, who monitors and encourages appropriate conduct all year long.

The Kitchen God, named Zao Jun or Zao Shen (Master of the Stove), is the most important of the many domestic gods that protect the home and family. Many Chinese believe that on the twenty-third day of the twelfth lunar month, just days before the Chinese New Year, the Kitchen God visits heaven to report to the Jade Emperor on every household's activities during the year. Then the emperor rewards or punishes families based on the Kitchen God's annual report.

The most popular origin story of the Kitchen God dates to the second century BC. Originally a mortal named Zhang Lang, he left his virtuous wife for a younger woman. As punishment for his adultery, the heavens blinded him whereupon his young lover abandoned him, and he was left to beg door to door for food. He came upon the home of his former wife without realizing it. She took pity on him and fed him well while he told his sad story. She told him to open his eyes and as he gazed upon his former wife's face, his vision was miraculously restored.

Overcome with shame, he threw himself into the kitchen hearth, unaware it was lit. All that was saved was one of his legs, which the devoted woman placed on a shrine above the fireplace, hence, Zhang Lang's association with the hearth. To this day in China, fire pokers are often called Zhang Lang's leg.

A second tale claims Zhang Lang was so poor he had to sell his wife; then unwittingly he became a servant in the home of her new husband. Once again, his kind-hearted wife felt sorry for him and baked him a cake filled with money. He failed to notice the hidden gift, sold the cake for a pittance, and upon realizing his mistake, took his own life.

The Heavens took pity on Zhang Lang and spared him the life of a *jiangshi*, or hopping vampire, the fate that befalls those that commit suicide based on Chinese folklore. The Chinese word *jiang* means "stiff." *Jiangshi* are thought to be so stiff they cannot bend their bodies, so they must move around by hopping while keeping their arms outstretched for balance. The hopping vampires hunt at night, killing living creatures to absorb their qi.

The legend of hopping vampires comes from the ancient practice of transporting a corpse over a thousand *li* (ancient Chinese mile). Often relatives of a person who died far from home couldn't afford a vehicle to transport the deceased; however, being buried away from home was considered a cruelty. So, to transport the bodies back home, corpses were arranged upright, single file and attached to long bamboo poles, while two men carried the poles on their shoulders at either end. When the bamboo poles flexed, the dead bodies appeared to be hopping up and down in unison.

Lucky for Zhang Lang, the Jade Emperor proclaimed that he had surely suffered through life's many lessons and earned the gift of all knowing and all seeing. I'd say Zhang got a good deal—better a spy than a hopping vampire.

The Nanyuan Teahouse featured two shrines to the Kitchen God: one traditional and a modern one that would make Elvis proud. The first shrine consisted of a simple porcelain statute of a man with a long black beard sitting atop a horizontal, wooden beam. A red curtain hung above the figure, candles and fruit offerings covered the beam, and lines of Chinese characters decorated the wall on either side of the shrine.

The second shrine was much more modern, flamboyant, and a bit garish. It was the perfect décor for any Chinese restaurant in Las Vegas but seemed rather out of place in the venerable teahouse. The elaborate plastic shrine featured a small, model of a temple with dramatic eaves, a fenced balcony, and ruffled gold curtains. In the center of the balcony stood a large, extremely colorful statue of the Kitchen God surrounded by electric candles and oranges.

In most Chinese homes, the Kitchen God is represented by a simple paper image which is hung next to the stove for a year. Roughly a week before the New Year, the image is burned and the ashes ascend to the Jade Emperor in heaven. Those with a permanent shrine or wooden plaque burn joss paper (decorative paper offerings for spirits) every year.

In my opinion, the Chinese have the right idea with a full-time, good-behavior informant (our seasonal Elf on the Shelf just doesn't get the job done).

When judgement day is upon us, it appears everyone gets a bit nervous. Many Chinese families have been known to smear the Kitchen God's mouth with honey or molasses—to sugar-coat his tongue and entice a positive report. Other families dip the paper deity in alcohol to sweeten the flames. Then, on New Year's

Eve, a new portrait of the Kitchen God is placed next to the stove for yet another year of snooping.

One of my strongest memories of Tongli is of two tiny old ladies, each probably less than five feet tall, sharing a single umbrella as they hobbled down an ancient cobblestone path alongside a canal flanked by willow trees. I couldn't help but think of the story of the golden lotus. Legend tells of a young girl who lost a toe and the king who searched the land for the tiny "lotus shoe" that could fit her; a darker version of the tale of Cinderella and the glass slipper and the cruel tradition of foot binding, unique only to China.

Emperor Li Yu of the Southern Tang dynasty is said to have created a large, golden lotus decorated with jewels for his favorite concubine, Yao Niang. He then asked her to bind her feet in white silk in the shape of a crescent moon and perform a ballet on the points of her toes atop the golden lotus platform. Her gracefulness drew envy and started a foot-binding epidemic, which started with wealthy, noble women but soon spread throughout the country.

The barbaric process began between the ages of four and nine. The practice involved curling the toes of each foot under, pressing down with extreme force, and squeezing the feet into tiny shoes until the toes broke. The broken toes were held against the soles of the feet with bandages, which were regularly tightened, until the arch of the foot broke as well. The perfectly bound foot (or golden lotus) was three Chinese inches (around four inches or ten centimeters in Western dimensions) or smaller, the larger "silver lotuses" were four Chinese inches, and the "iron lotuses" were five Chinese inches.

The smaller a woman's bound feet, the more likely she was to have a prestigious marriage; therefore, foot binding became a prerequisite for finding a husband. In poor households, the eldest daughter would bind her feet while her younger sisters trained to be her handmaids, all in the hope of joining a wealthy family.

Millions of women bound their feet to become more desirable to men, many of whom found a woman's feet to be the most sensual part of her body and an erotic symbol of femininity. Those women with bound feet were said to have a lotus gait, characterized by walking on their heels, taking small steps, and swaying as they walked.

By the nineteenth century, it was estimated that 40 to 50 percent of Chinese women had bound feet, and among upper class Han Chinese women, the figure was almost 100 percent. By the twentieth century, a very small percentage of young girls had bound feet. By 1912, regional governments were sending inspectors to fine women for binding their feet. Starting in 1949, the communist regime began to harshly criticize the custom. These days, foot binding is thankfully a thing of the past; the last reported foot binding being in 1957.

As much as I admire the Chinese for continuing to adhere to time-honored traditions, foot binding is one practice I'm very glad has ceased to exist. I could relate to the Chinese women's desperation to improve their social status with a beneficial marriage as I was bound and determined to change my social status by becoming a mother.

As a woman and a future mother to a Chinese girl, learning about this inhumane aspect of China's history was very upsetting and difficult to fathom. I was thankful my future daughter would never have to experience this sort of self-abuse and injustice in the name of beauty and social status. Puberty, braces, teenage cliques, and high heels are bad enough.

After exploring nearly every inch of Tongli, my feet hurt from walking, my back hurt from carrying a growing number of souvenirs, and most of all my hands hurt from scribbling nonstop in my journal. As I began to limp, I was flooded with memories of the sharp pain, deep soreness, and many intense side effects from over a year of taking fertility drugs.

Back in the day, when I was a fertility drug junkie, willing to ingest or inject any and all fertility boosting medications in the desperate hopes of a baby, our master bathroom looked like a meth lab. The bathroom counter was completely covered with a medication calendar, alcohol wipes, sterile water, bottles of powder, vials of liquid, and a wide variety of needles of varying lengths and thicknesses (some for mixing and others for injecting medication).

One of the drugs I was prescribed was made from the purified urine of postmenopausal Italian nuns, since postmenopausal women excrete large amounts of an egg growth stimulating hormone in their pee. I was also given a medication produced from the ovaries of Chinese hamsters. Chinese hamster ovary, or CHO, cells are relatively easy to grow, and the genes were being used for anticancer drugs, hemophiliac medicine, and psoriasis treatments.

Yep, that's correct, I got shot up with virginal pee and hamster ovarian cells, all in the name of motherhood—and still didn't have a baby.

After lunch, I limped back through the official entrance gates of Tongli. In 1982, Tongli was listed for protection as a standard provincial town of cultural interest in Jiangsu Province. Sadly, this once quaint and picturesque water town had already become a crowded tourist destination with an entrance fee of one hundred yuan (sixteen dollars). Some of its historical and cultural value has been lost to tacky souvenir shops, overbearing street vendors, and satellite dishes, but it would take a lot more modernization before Tongli loses all its rural, small-town charm.

After walking throughout Tongli, I was definitely ready for the taxi ride to Shanghai, but my current discomfort still paled in comparison to the vivid memories of my husband injecting hormones into my ass.

As we drove to Shanghai, Leo told us a fascinating story about the legendary Empress Dowager Cixi, who was nothing if not determined and a bit desperate—like me.

Is it possible to want something too much? Go too far to achieve a goal? Is the desire worth the risks? Even if it's as noble a dream as motherhood? My desperation to have a child caused me to risk my own physical and mental health, my marriage, and my personal finances, which in a bizarre way made me feel connected to the ruthlessly determined Empress Dowager Cixi.

I was greatly intrigued by this woman, who clawed and pushed her way to a high position, formidable power, and massive wealth—eventually making the Summer Palace in Beijng her home. The cunning Cixi did many questionable things to get the Xi'anfeng Emperor's attention, become his favorite concubine, and ultimately rise to power as an empress. While I didn't approve of her rather maniacal methods, I admired her tenacity and was inspired by her determination.

According to Leo, in 1851, at the age of sixteen, Cixi participated in the selection of concubines for the Xi'anfeng

Emperor alongside sixty other candidates and placed in the sixth rank of consorts. Legend has it she paid eunuchs for information on the emperor's location, so that they could "casually" cross paths and he could "overhear" her singing.

"The emperor gave Cixi a beautiful white cat that made the other concubines jealous," Leo said. "One day, Cixi found the cat boiled to death in a pot. Later, when she became empress, she found the concubine who did it and boiled her in a pot."

Cixi provided the first and only surviving son for the royal family in 1856. However, the emperor already had a wife, the Empress Ci'an. By her son's first birthday, Cixi was elevated to a third rank consort, second only to the empress. Unlike other women in the imperial household, Cixi was known for her ability to read and write Chinese. She became well informed about state affairs and the art of governing and became an aide to the ailing emperor. Upon the emperor's death, Cixi, as the highest ranked consort and the Emperor's widow were both named Empresses Dowager (the title given to a mother or widow of a Chinese emperor). The Empress Dowager Ci'an became known as the Empress of the East, while Cixi was called the Empress of the West.

According to legend, as he lay upon his death-bed, the emperor, who knew how power-hungry and ruthless Cixi could be, gave his wife an order that allowed her to kill Cixi if she tried to kill her first. "After the emperor's death," Leo explained, "the East Empress fell ill, and Cixi saw a golden opportunity. The only cure for what ailed Ci'an was phoenix meat, and since the phoenix was a symbol of the empress herself, Cixi cut some meat off her leg to save her. The phoenix meat cured the East Empress and made Cixi look good and kind. However, Cixi then gave the East Empress poisoned cookies. After her death, Cixi took over and became a very powerful empress."

Whether a despot responsible for the fall of the Qing dynasty, a talented woman desperate to change her fate, or a victim of factors beyond her command, Cixi effectively controlled the Chinese government for forty-seven years, from 1861 until her death in 1908. Upon her death, the court was left in shambles.

Whether history chooses to vilify or glorify Cixi, I found the Empress Dowager Cixi's shrewdness in some degree commendable. She didn't let anything stand in the way of her goals, just as I would have done almost anything (except bribing, boiling, or poisoning anyone) to have a child. I applauded her determination, not her methods.

I have to admit that I truly share the iron-clad will of the Empress Dowager Cixi—at least in this one small regard.

14

BRIGHT LIGHTS—BIG CITY

In a word, Shanghai was *overwhelming*. The words *crowded*, *intense*, and *fast-paced* would have been gross understatements. The dizzying energy of the thriving metropolis was palpable. Shanghai made New York City and Los Angeles look like sleepy country towns.

If the dense population of Beijing made me feel like a single ant navigating through a supercolony, the insane pace of Shanghai made me feel like a hamster stuck in a ball, frantically trying to get out of the way and not get run over.

Currently, China, at 1.37 billion people, is only slightly ahead of India, at 1.29 billion people, for the title of world's highest population. Shanghai used to be the most populated city in the world but is now ranked third, at 24.5 million people, behind Tokyo (38 million) and Dehli (26.4 million). As crowded as Shanghai was, I couldn't fathom life in Delhi or Tokyo. It's inconceivable.

The old concept of *duozi-duofu* or "more children, more happiness" led to an explosive expansion of the population of China, which in turn strained the country's economy, threatened resources, and affected the general quality of life. Faced with the threat of starvation, many believed the country had no choice but to impose population control measures, namely the one-child policy in 1979 and the promotion of the concept "less children, better quality."

As the country continues to struggle with population issues, the effects on the quality and pace of life, especially in major cities like Shanghai, were sobering. Living in Shanghai seemed to me like living in a K-Pop music video (complete with ridiculous numbers of extremely perky Asian teens) or being trapped in a live-action version of the video game *Street Fighter*.

As we ventured into the melee that is the Nanjing Road Pedestrian Mall, with neon lights, digital billboards and live-action displays that rival the world-renowned Times Square in New York City, I feared the intense visual stimulation might induce a seizure. Meanwhile Chris said, "I feel like I'm in a staring contest with the Hypno-Toad" (from the animated series *Futurama*).

The pedestrian mall is three and a half miles long (5.5 km) and packed with more than six hundred shops. Nanjing Road had it all: fast food restaurants; upscale shops like Tiffany's, Mont Blanc, and Dunhill; open-air bars and fancy eateries; giant department stores; dozens of traditional Chinese stores; and enormous souvenir shops. Street performers, musicians, and peddlers wandered about amongst abstract sculptures and modern-art installations.

Navigating through the staggering number of moving bodies on Nanjing Road was beyond intimidating, so a trackless sightseeing train was available for anyone too overwhelmed to fight through the huge crowds. Bravely walking along the pedestrian mall, I felt like I had unwillingly joined a hive of bees, constantly buzzing, perpetually in motion, and swarming in and out of stores in mindless droves.

Shanghai has been called the Paris of the East, for it is truly a consumer's paradise. As China's style capital and most cosmopolitan city, Shanghai caters to serious shopping addicts with a lot of energy, patience, and platinum credit cards.

I am not a fashionista and couldn't care less about brand names. As a writer, I spend most of my time at home, often wearing the same comfortable yoga pants and hoodie for several days in a row. I have a perpetual ponytail and own way too many baseball caps. I figure my dogs don't care if I dress up or wear make-up and if my computer doesn't care for my laid-back attire it hasn't yet voiced its negative opinion. As for Chris, he's gotten used to me "borrowing" his T-shirts.

I like comfortable, sensible clothes and own one pair of simple, black heels for weddings and holiday parties. (I'm embarrassed to admit that I live in rubbery Crocs shoes and a decade-old pair of Dansko clogs). I shop at discount, consignment, and thrift stores and if I feel like splurging, I go to Target. Every month, I drool over the Athleta catalog but never order anything. I avoid the mall like the plague and don't know the first thing about designers or current styles. Chris swears I'm a purse addict, but in truth I hate purses and only continue to shop for handbags due to an unending quest to find the smallest, but most functional, purse in the known universe.

Suffice it to say, as a work-from-home, practical tomboy who hates to shop (my penchant for folk art being the one exception), I was very much out of my element in Shanghai, and very much overwhelmed.

After getting trapped on the seventh floor of an enormous department store, because all the down elevators were full, our first evening in Shanghai failed to improve. Mind you, this was the end of our trip when we were running on empty and running out of money. We were not only tired and broke, we were navigating the most overstimulating and overwhelming city we would experience on this trip. What we needed more than anything was some downtime to connect. We longed for a quiet dinner together, some moments away from the chaos and commotion.

Flipping through our guidebook and finding what looked like a unique dining experience, I'd planned the perfect, romantic dinner. Our destination was Kathleen's 5, an upscale restaurant on the top floor of the Shanghai Art Museum. It had a glassed-in dining area and provided spectacular views of Renmin Gongyuan (People's Park).

We arrived with full appetites and high expectations only to learn that we needed a reservation (months ago) and that dinner with a view came with a price tag we couldn't afford. With empty stomachs and rotten moods, we continued to wander around People's Park. We had heard about a place named Barbarossa, an iconic Shanghai establishment with a Moroccan flavor on a boat at the edge of a lake. The restaurant, bar, and lounge offered three floors of food, cocktails, hookahs, music, and a serene, oasis atmosphere. Though fiercely determined, practically starving, and fighting back tears of frustration, we never found Barbarossa. We circled around People's Park two times, we asked directions from a guard who rolled his eyes and pointed to indicate the closeness of the nightclub, and ultimately searched until the park closed. (The next day, we learned that Barbarossa was closed for renovations and that the lake was temporarily drained. If only we had searched for construction cranes and a mud hole.)

Chris and I had fallen in love again in this fascinating, vibrant country, and now our bond was being put to the test as we wandered around in the dark—starving, tired, and miserable. It was a credit to us and our marriage that we weren't on the verge of killing each other, which proved how far we'd come after conquering many tests of our relationship in the past several years. We had walked for miles, gotten completely lost in the dark in a foreign city, and didn't eat until nearly midnight, but we didn't take our frustration out on each other, we got through the disastrous date night, defeated but still a united front.

Exhausted, hungry, and cranky we returned to Nanjing Road completely downtrodden. We dined at the first restaurant we could find, a place called Babela's Kitchen. We ate Chinese pizza with chicken, ham, and sausage (all of which I removed), as well as, mushrooms, onions and peppers (all of which Chris removed) making the most of what we could order via randomly pointing. We noticed the Chinese ate their pizza with a fork and knife and sat far away from the uncivilized Americans eating with their hands.

After we left the restaurant, I vented my frustration over our epically failed romantic evening by stopping at a candy store and purchasing obscene amounts of Chinese candy. The candy store was larger than most American health-food markets and was completely packed with frantic shoppers (seemingly desperate but not entirely in need of a late-night sugar fix).

Like a spoiled and compulsive Veruca Salt, I braved the frenzied crowd around the ten-yuan bargain bin and impulsively purchased a large variety of mysterious cellophane bundles.

Even something as mundane as a bag of candy or a box of chocolate was beautifully packaged in China. The most popular design motif appeared to be 1920s Chinese, pin-up girls and images of Shanghai during its heyday in the Roaring Twenties.

As we walked back to our hotel around 1:00 a.m., we were approached by some rather unsavory characters trying to sell event tickets and knock-off merchandise. Once again, I was bombarded with "Hello, Lady." "Watches." "Sunglasses." "Hand Bags." "Hello, Pretty Lady." "You look. You like." And they didn't take *Bù Yào!* or "Not want" for an answer.

When Chris ventured out again alone to smoke a cigar (his chosen sympathy prize for the epic-fail evening), he was offered prostitutes and marijuana. The pimps took their job seriously. They presented display books with full color photos and bios for each "takeout girl."

They said, "make love, Chinese girl," as though the word *love* might exonerate the act of prostitution.

Chris got so frustrated after numerous failed attempts to discourage the overbearing pimps, that he began responding to them in Swedish. They, in turn, tried their best to counter with a bit of German, but eventually gave up and walked away in disgruntled defeat.

When Chris returned and told me what happened, his description of the brochure booklets for takeout girls made me think of the "brag books" sold at Walgreens. I had always envisioned the mini photo albums being used by grandmas to carry photographs of their precious grandkids to Bingo Night.

As I drifted off to sleep that night, after a rather exasperating first evening in Shanghai, I thought, "If we can manage traveling in fast-paced, chaotic China together, we can overcome any of life's challenges. After four years in the throes of infertility, what's a few crazy nights in Shanghai? Our marriage is strong, and we are resilient." Shanghai showed me that, or maybe I knew it all along . . . but forgot.

I completed my crash course in Buddhism at the Jade Buddha Temple. After a month in China, I'm proud to say that I could easily recognize the Four Heavenly Kings, Buddha's official protector (Wei Tuo), and Hotei (the Laughing Buddha).

In 1882, a temple was built to house two Buddha statues from Burma, carved entirely of jade. The temple was destroyed during the overthrow of the Qing dynasty, but the figures were saved. The new Jade Buddha Temple was built in 1928 as a home for the two statues and many other sacred Buddhist statues, paintings, and scriptures.

Every inch of the stunning Jade Buddha Temple was beautifully and symbolically decorated. Ornately carved wooden lanterns and embroidered silk banners hung from the ceilings, while short, red stools for praying covered the floors. Tiny roof guardians, mystical dragons, and protective fish tiles lined the peaked eaves of the temple roofs. In the courtyard, small citrus and bonsai trees were adorned with red ribbons and covered with coins. The heavy scents of fresh flower bouquets, numerous offerings of oranges and candle and incense smoke filled the air. Together with the huge crowd of visitors, it was a bit stifling.

A large hollow wooden fish sat in the temple courtyard. When hit with a mallet, it made a deep sound (like a Chinese foghorn). They rang the fish bell to ke p the monks on task. According to our Shanghai guide, Daisy, a fish was given the important job of keeping the monks focused because it never closes its eyes.

Also, in the temple were the famed Sitting Buddha and Recumbent Buddha. They were both carved from exotic, white jade. The Sitting Buddha was encrusted with agate and emerald and depicted Buddha at the moment of his enlightenment. The Recumbent Buddha portrayed Buddha in a peaceful pose known as the lucky repose that represents the deity's attainment of nirvana.

It's no coincidence that the character for *emperor* (丰) is very similar to the character for *jade* (玉) since the souls of emperors are said to live within jade. The best jade comes from Australia, but white jade, which is very rare and extremely expensive, is the pride of China. It's not an overstatement that ancient kingdoms in China started wars over precious pieces of jade.

In general, images of Buddha feature large hands, feet, and ears. The Chinese believe that being born with big ears, like Buddha, is good luck. Sadly, Americans don't share this notion, so when I was born with big ears that stuck straight out from the sides of my head, my father intervened. I spent the summer after second grade with a cast around my head to pin my ears back. Even now, after having had work done, the tops of my ears round outward—in a determined effort to remain lucky.

Roughly 80 percent of the residents of Shanghai practice Buddhism, and the elderly, female Buddhists of Shanghai were super hard-core! They pushed through crowds of people as if they owned the place and were on a mission from Buddha. They were determined that their prayers be heard, and nothing was going to stop them, not hordes of tourists or Mara, the demon that tempted Prince Siddhartha herself.

The single-minded old ladies prayed to the four directions, turning in a clockwise circle, holding bundles of incense in both hands. They prayed with five parts: two legs, two hands, and one head, bowing toward the earth.

I thought about beseeching the Jade Buddha for the gift of motherhood; but in this crowded temple full of determined and downright intense Buddhists, I felt I hadn't yet earned the right—so I simply made a donation.

One afternoon we took a stroll along the Bund to view the international architecture and famous skyline of Shanghai.

The Bund is a mile-long waterfront promenade within the former Shanghai International Settlement, which runs alongside the west bank of the Huangpu River. The views of the modern skyscrapers in the Pudong District on the opposite bank are spectacular.

Shanghai's prime location on the Yangtze River Delta made it a major trading port in imperial China, and its huge economic potential led to conflict over control of the city in the nineteenth century. The British were the first foreigners to have access to Shanghai. After the First Opium War, British consuls and merchants settled in the city. Soon after the Americans and French established concessions. After the First Sino-Japanese War, Japan also became a foreign power in Shangai, and they even occupied the city during World War II. Throughout the twentieth century, the Bund developed into the main financial center of east Asia.

"At one time, there were French, British, and American international concessions with different currencies, languages, and technology," Daisy said. "They were like small countries within the larger country of China. The Chinese learned about balconies and elevators from the foreigners."

The Bund's "museum of world architecture" includes dozens of historical structures in various styles, including Gothic, Baroque, Roman, Renaissance, and Neoclassical, that once housed banks and trading houses from Great Britain, France, and the United States, to name a few. In addition, Russian and British consulates, the *North China Daily News,* and the Shanghai Club were located on the legendary avenue.

Of all the exquisite and historic buildings on the Bund, I was most fascinated by the Peace Hotel. As I stepped into its grand lobby, I felt like I had been transported to the Shanghai of the 1920s; the pin-up girls on my souvenir boxes of chocolate roared back to life, and I felt like I was literally walking through history.

The hotel was once known as the Number One Mansion in the Far East for its distinctive green copper roof, white Italian marble floors, priceless glass chandeliers, Art Deco details, and renowned Old Jazz Bar. During its famously decadent heyday from the 1920s to the 1930s, international jet-setters and local socialites frequented costume parties, grand balls, and concerts held at the hotel. On more than one occasion, the sometimes-scandalous events brought the police and made newspaper headlines.

By far the biggest fashion trend in China during the 1920s was the qiapao. It's been said that the qiapao is to China what the kimono is to Japan and the sari is to India. Known in the south as a cheongsam, the qiapao, which literally means "banner dress," refers to the embroidered silk gowns worn by Manchu women of the Banner class, army regiments of the Qing dynasty. Upon establishment of the Qing dynasty in 1644, the upper-class Han women were forced to adopt the dress, but the style saw its true heyday in the 1920s and 1930s among the socialites of Shanghai.

Over time, the qipao progressed from wide, loose, and knee-length to long and form-fitting, with revealing thigh-high side slits. During the Cultural Revolution (1966-1976), the qipao was considered bourgeois and women traded them in for blue cotton pantsuits, known in the West as Mao suits.

I tried desperately to stuff myself into a gorgeous indigo qipao in a vintage store in the French Concession area. Alas, the traditional Chinese fashion doesn't accommodate a 34-D bust. Sadly, my figure is more of a 1950s hourglass than a 1920s toothpick. All was not lost, as I found a child's red, embroidered silk jacket, perfect for all Chinese festivals and holidays, and couldn't have been happier (although I teared up a bit as the saleswoman wrapped the jacket in plastic, for future use).

Most of the historic mansions in the former French Concession were hidden behind huge hedges and rows of trees. However, those ancient villas that were visible were a sad sight. The vast majority of the once-majestic homes in the French Concession area were completely run down, if not utterly destroyed, by modernization and time. Once-charming, lavish estate homes were now subdivided and overrun by multiple tenants, all of whom dumped their trash in the formerly manicured courtyards and displayed their national flags across the ornate balconies.

The Bund is also known as Lovers' Street. Many old apartments in Shanghai were so small they only had communal areas. (They didn't even have kitchens or bathrooms.) So lovers would head to the Bund to get busy on top of an old flood prevention wall.

The flood wall was replaced in the 1990s with a more efficient and decorative wall but was still known as the Lovers' Wall. The mile-long wall of colored brick and granite has a viewing deck with thirty-two semi-circle balconies as well as pavilions, benches, and unique murals made of flowers.

It seemed the Bund's popular Lovers' Wall was also *the* place to take a photo with your sweetheart, bestie, coworkers, tour group, or family—and a blonde, American "celebrity." I was asked to join in no less than seven photographs with Asian tourists.

I stood in the middle of a group of high school students on a field trip (their teacher even handed me the school flag to hold), while numerous teachers, chaperones, and random passersby took photos. I was asked to join a wedding party photo and was placed in between the bride and groom. I was also featured in the center of a giggly group of young, Korean girls wearing Hello Kitty headbands. But my favorite photo was with a tiny, old man who stood next to me, holding onto my arm with one hand while he reached up above my shoulder with his other hand to accentuate our extreme height difference.

Chris and I noticed an interesting theme amongst the Asian tourists taking travel photos. They all—young or old; Chinese, Korean, or Japanese; in groups or individuals—made the peace or victory sign. According to Daisy, the raised index and middle fingers in a V shape, with the palm out, is considered a Y by Asians and stands for Yeah!

Perhaps the sign's earliest roots come from Japanese Manga. Also, the Japanese began to emulate the signature peace sign of American figure skater, Janet Lynn, after she fell during her performance at the 1972 Olympics in Japan but kept a positive attitude, which the Japanese greatly admired.

Possibly the largest influence on the V sign epidemic in east Asia was Japanese singer Jun Inoue of The Spiders. Inoue was the celebrity spokesmodel for Konica cameras and flashed a spontaneous V sign during the filming of a Konica commercial in 1972. The mass production of cameras led to an influx of magazines for girls and women, featuring the aesthetics of *kawaii*, or the culture based on superficial cuteness, which led to an explosion of the V sign on social media.

Whatever their personal reason for flashing the Y or V sign, every single Asian tourist—from packs of teenagers to groups of businessmen to toddlers on a family vacation—displayed the Y symbol in their photos. It was surreal to witness such an intrinsic aspect of Asian culture that is tantamount to American photographers insisting that everyone say cheese or adding bunny ears to your brother—it's second nature.

Our stroll along the Bund was a perfect introduction to Shanghai's international background and mix of old and new. Ancient Shanghai was represented by historic, European, Beaux-Arts-style buildings on the west side and modern Shanghai glowing with neon skyscrapers on the east side of the Huangpu River.

According to Daisy, the locals have a saying that You haven't seen Shanghai if you haven't seen the Bund, and the Bund's appeal was tremendous. But for the baby boomers of Shanghai, the Bund will always be a place for romance (and a sentimental make-out spot).

One night, we wandered past a blur of moving bodies, flashing lights, and general madness on the Nanjing Road pedestrian mall until we found our old, familiar friend: the Chinese convenience store.

Convenience stores had become our nightly oasis away from the noise, energy, and chaos. During each visit, we felt like kids let loose in a toy store with our birthday money from Grandma. The excitement was nearly palpable as we hunted for random souvenirs and bizarre snacks among the shelves stocked with unfamiliar products in exotic, colorful packaging. We couldn't decipher the Chinese characters on the food and drink labels, so whatever we bought was a complete mystery.

We would hurry back to our hotel room with our loot and dump our treasures on the bed, like kids with party favor bags after a slumber party. Then, with our goodies arrayed, we would share snacks, pass drinks back and forth, and marvel over our curiosities.

We had great fun tricking and double dog daring each other to be the first to try exotic Chinese delicacies and liquors.

One of us would say, "Try this drink; it's awesome, I swear." Then the other one would gag and sputter, "You tricked me; it's like swallowing the sun!"

Many times, we thought we had purchased something sweet only to take a bite and discover something savory. A round white bun could be filled with sweet red bean paste or cabbage and pork. Even the pink bun, which appeared to be dusted with powdered sugar, turned out to be a shrimp ball. One time, we thought we were buying alcohol, only to learn we had purchased iced tea. Our convenience store purchases were always a gamble, but an entertaining one (that usually ended in trading kisses for bravery).

On that particular night we purchased our standard comfort items: local fire water and China's version of Twinkies. We chose a variety pack of mini bottles of China's legendary *baijiu* or clear liquor. Based on China's massive population, baijiu is the world's most highly consumed alcohol, although few Westerners can tolerate it. Baijiu has a distinct savory, strong-as-hell flavor, which legendary American newsman Dan Rather described as "liquid razor blades." Often referred to as Chinese vodka, baijiu is mainly distilled from sorghum and rice, then fermented with yeast and sugar. The most famous and expensive Maotai baijiu is refined seven times and matured for at least three years, gaining a potency of 40 to 55 percent alcohol. Maotai is credited with smoothing Chinese-American relations during a meeting between Mao Zedong and Richard Nixon with only three cups.

The convenience store clerk, who was a college student eager to practice his English, greatly approved of our baijiu variety pack purchase and told us "Have fun, but good luck, you will need some. Very strong stuff."

Returning to the Central Hotel, we enjoyed a relaxing night of baijiu, "Twinkies," and local television. There were only two English language channels to choose from, so we watched *Allan Quartermain and the Lost City of Gold* out of sheer desperation. The campy 1980s flick was an obvious, poor quality, knock-off of the Indiana Jones series. The one-star movie featured Sharon Stone as an archeologist. She was nominated for a Golden Raspberry Award for worst actress but lost to Madonna for *Who's that Girl*. Sadly, this was the best of our options, when up against *American Ninja 3*.

After a few shots of baijiu, with a taste combination of rotten papaya, aged Roequefort cheese, and sweaty socks, James Earl Jones' portrayal of a Zulu warrior became much more entertaining.

I wondered if the Chinese saying "First we must taste the bitter things so that we may recognize the sweet" was inspired by baijiu, since just about anything would taste better by comparison. Then again, after drinking baijiu, your taste buds become so scorched and your brain so discombobulated, you might feel brave enough to eat a scorpion on a stick or dare I say a donkey penis. Or perhaps it's simply a beautiful and apt proverb about the ups and downs of life, the whims of time and the lessons learned from a difficult journey. In the end, earned achievements after a long struggle bring more appreciation and happiness than easy gains—like the long road to motherhood for instance. Or maybe, I was just drunk on Chinese liquid courage.

Whatever the reason, it was becoming clear that China, or in that moment its baijiu, had gone to my head and heart. Unlike with previous trips after pregnancy failures and losses, where we returned rested and a bit more relaxed, but still tethered to our pain, in China, we finally let go and put our misfortunes in the past. I felt rejuvenated and reawakened. I was no longer afraid to live boldly and with hope for the future. As Buddha once said, "We, ourselves, must walk the path, live joyfully, and have faith, for you are the master."

15

THE PEN RUNS DRY

One morning, with the promise of a reprieve from the rain, we headed to the Oriental Pearl Tower for a panoramic view of Shanghai. Completed in 1994, the tower was the tallest structure in China until 2007 and featured eleven spheres of various sizes linked by three giant columns. The enormous pillar looked like the Eiffel Tower with bubbles and reminded me of typical images from 1970s sci-fi flicks, possibly a death ray, tractor beam, or anal probe. The unique tower design was easy to spot any time of day, but the multi-sequenced LED lights really made the tower sparkle at night. "Beam me up, Scotty!"

The tower's design was rumored to be an homage to the Tang dynasty poem "Pipa Song" by Bai Juyi. It's about the tinkling sound made by a pipa instrument, "like pearls, big and small, falling on a jade plate." It's a fair comparison since the tower of various sized orbs was surrounded by a lush, green park.

Visitors, up to fifty at a time, traveled to the top of the tower in double-decker elevators at a rate of twenty-three feet (seven meters) per second for the rapid quarter-mile ascent. The tower has fifteen observation levels. The highest, known as the Space

Module, is 1,148 feet (350 meters). Sadly, even on a sunny day it was difficult to see much of anything through the smog.

In addition to serving the city with upward of ten radio and TV channels, the Oriental Pearl also features a revolving restaurant (one of six in Shanghai and the highest in Asia) and a twenty-room Space Hotel (for those who want to experience life like *The Jetsons*). Our guide, Daisy, told us many Chinese tourists visit the Oriental Pearl Tower simply to use the restroom. "They go to the tower just to say that they've used the toilet at the top of the world."

The highlight for us was the Shanghai Municipal History Museum, which was formerly located in the tower's pedestal. The small but captivating museum featured art, culture, and industrialization scenes and models from one hundred years of Shanghai's history, including a teahouse, a Chinese pharmacy, and traditional homes. The museum's oldest relics were six thousand years old and included a cannon from the first Opium War, an elaborate sedan wedding chair, and two bronze guardian lions that had once stood watch over the banks along the Bund.

As we left the Oriental Pearl Tower and strolled toward the Yuyuan Garden and Market, we came across an incredible sculptured gate shaped like a stone dragon at the entrance to the Dragon Gate Mall. The dragon gate had a shallow-river flowing across its arched backside and a machine that filled the tunnel under its belly with smoke. The huge dragon was reaching for a giant stone pearl in the center of a beautiful manicured flower bed.

We watched as a large Asian family posed for a photo together under the bridge. As they all began to flash the standard V sign, the smoke machine turned on and the elderly matriarch of the family started wailing and flailing her arms about like she was banishing the devil. Whereupon her grandkids started falling over from laughter and kept trying to push their grandmother back under the bridge. When we left, grandma was still sitting resolutely on a park bench, swatting at her family members with her purse and refusing to budge.

Yu in Chinese means "joyful," a befitting name for the Yuyuan Garden, known as the Garden of Happiness, which was surprisingly tranquil, even though it borders the chaotic Yuyuan Market.

The classical garden was begun in 1559 by Ming dynasty official Pan Yunduan as a gift for his aging father, the minister Pan En. He began the project after failing one of his imperial exams, but his successful appointment as governor of Sichuan postponed construction nearly twenty years, until 1577. Sadly, while the garden was the grandest of its era in Shanghai, the expense helped to financially ruin the Pan family.

The beautifully restored, five-acre garden was filled with grand halls, elegant pavilions, massive rockeries, zigzag bridges, moon-shaped gates, and several ponds. The six scenic areas of the garden were separated by "dragon walls" with an undulating backbone of grey tiles and giant, metal dragon heads on both sides of each entrance gate. The dragons had only four claws, unlike the imperial five-clawed dragons, so as not to anger the emperor.

Much of the charm of the Yuyuan Garden was in the details. Chris and I had an adventure hunting for the tiny clay sculptures, works of calligraphy, painted and carved bricks, and poetic inscriptions hidden throughout the enchanting garden.

I spent the better part of an hour feeding several hundred koi fish swimming in a series of large, rock-lined, green pools. The main pond was literally teaming with bright orange ones, white ones, and even calico-patterned ones. Many of the fish were enormous, and they were swarming over each other several fish deep, like a fast-moving lava flow. The fish performed all sorts of entertaining calisthenics to reach the top of the heap.

I took off my shoes, sat on a boulder, and dangled my bare feet over the pond, whereupon, hundreds of fish sucked on my toes. The scandalous removal of my shoes and uncontrollable giggling drew lots of attention. Numerous people took my photo and several children came and joined me (but sadly their legs were too short for the fish to nibble at their toes).

I felt like the Pied Piper of China, doling out handfuls of fish food to my wide-eyed following of young koi fish enthusiasts (in lieu of hypnotized German children or rats).

As I sat feeding the fish in the Yuyuan Garden, I couldn't help but think of our tiny koi pond in Colorado, where I spent numerous hours attempting to calm my nerves and meditate during the many trials of infertility treatments.

I remember one day quite vividly. After our first IVF attempt, I was too scared to take a slightly unreliable home pregnancy test, so I opted for an official pregnancy test from my doctor.

We were on pins and needles waiting for that phone call, so we sought distraction and solace in the backyard. While I pretended to relax in the hammock, Chris puttered around the pond, checking filters, tending to plants, and feeding fish. It was a beautiful afternoon and my anxiety might have begun to fade, just a little . . . if my husband's cellphone had not begun to ring. Just one look at his face and the world went cold and dark.

I ran sobbing into the house and collapsed on the living room floor. My heart ached, it hurt to breathe, and I felt completely lost from utter shock and disbelief.

That pain of failure paled in comparison to the anguish we suffered upon learning that the fragile life we created after our second IVF attempt hadn't developed a heartbeat. As I lay on a frigid and sterile examination table and the doctor told us our baby was no longer viable and needed to be surgically removed, I was reduced to nothingness and a wheelchair. I had lost all hope and desire to live.

But on that day in China I allowed myself only a moment of sad reflection. As the cool rain abated and the warm sunshine broke through the clouds, I sat surrounded by happy children. I took a deep breath, kept my center, and left my heartache in the past. Traveling to a foreign land had brought me back to life, strengthened my body and mind, and boosted my hope for a bright future. I was on a new path, away from darkness and into light.

After my pleasant hour spent feeding fish together with several children, I thought it befitting to purchase a fish charm, in hopes of a continuation of marital harmony and a future abundance of children. I found a talisman consisting of two matching halves of a wooden fish, painted red and attached to a silk cord. Together, the two pieces make a perfect koi fish (a symbol of unity since they swim in pairs), but when separated you can see images of children hidden inside.

I found this perfect fish charm at the ancient Yuyuan Market. The market was in the center of Nan Shi, the traditional name for the old, Chinese part of Shanghai. Once a Chinese-only walled enclave, when Shanghai was divided into foreign concessions, the Nan Shi walls dated from the sixteenth century. The old city walls were torn down in 1912, but a small piece of the original wall served as an entrance to the market on Renmin Road. The bazaar looked like a perfectly manufactured, Hollywood movie set. However, the buildings were authentic, more than a hundred years old and beautifully refurbished.

Centuries ago, the City God Temple, built in the fifteenth century, was the only thing in Nan Shi. But as the number of worshippers increased, so did the number of businesses, including pawn shops, banks, gold and silver stores, teahouses, and theaters. Now the area is home to a lively market featuring traditional Chinese art, antiques, clothing, food, and random junk.

We watched an elderly man at work on an ink-and-wash painting of a landscape. The artist worked incredibly fast, not only using bamboo brushes but also his hands. He used the sides of his palms and fingertips to create clouds and waterfalls and for blending and softening lines. It was mesmerizing. If I had watched long enough, I think I might have entered a trance, but he finished his masterpiece in less than five minutes. I purchased the small landscape for fourteen dollars; I thought it would make a lovely print for a baby nursery.

Next, I bought a tiny bottle with Chinese inner painting after watching a young artist, maybe fifteen-years-old, at work in the Yuyuan Market square. Somehow, the teenager managed to paint pictures and calligraphy on the inside surface of glass bottles by feeding a small brush through the neck of the bottle. To paint inside the delicate bottles, the young artist had to paint backwards, use very precise strokes, and have the concentration of a brain surgeon or a sword swallower. Inside painted bottles were originally used to hold snuff as early as the 1820s; though, I can't imagine filling the bottles, which are also works of art, with dark, ground tobacco.

I chose one of the smallest bottles, roughly four inches tall with the most intricate design of a pair of Asian cranes in a tree filled with cherry blossoms, as testament to the incredible artform. I watched as the artist painted my name in Chinese characters inside the tiny bottle. He told me that *ni* means "pretty" and *na* means "lady," but I'm fairly certain he just wanted a fat tip. Based on my research *ni* means "you" and *na* means "that," "then," or "take," but I gave him a nice tip for his artistic ability and charming attempt at flattery.

When traveling, there's nothing more uplifting than getting to know local children. Surely, there is no better way to understand, appreciate, and completely fall in love with another culture than interplay with its endearing youth.

I had already gained invaluable cultural insights from the variety of inquisitive youth I'd encountered so far in China, including a patty-cake partner, a young folk-song-singing guide, kindred koi fish enthusiasts, a flirtatious young artist, and fellow dancers (both teenaged minority and pint-sized hip hop dancers I was soon to meet). With this in mind, we spent an entertaining hour at the Shanghai Children's Palace, a youth center for the study of Chinese arts, dance, music, and calligraphy, as well as, math, science, and technology.

After the revolution of 1949, children's palaces were started all over China to provide childcare for children of working parents in the new Communist system. Shanghai's Children's Palace was established in 1953 by Song Qingling, the wife of political leader Dr. Sun Yat-sen. It was housed in the former private villa of an English merchant. The extravagant estate, known as the Marble Mansion, was built in 1924 and featured marble-lined hallways, wide curving staircases, and a front hall complete with ornate fireplaces, grand chandeliers, and stained-glass windows. In addition, the grounds held a science hall, recreation hall, small stage, and observatory.

When we visited, the walls of the mansion were filled with children's paintings, sketches, and lines of calligraphy. The rooms were filled with students learning extracurricular activities, including the ancient Chinese art of brushstroke painting and playing the erhu. The school offered more than a hundred clubs, for children ages four to sixteen, such as folk music, stamp collecting, reading, and astronomy, as well as various sports.

The after-school program operated on a shoestring budget; therefore, tourists were encouraged to visit (and support) the school. Our small donation not only helped fund various programs, it also gave us the unique opportunity to observe the lives of children growing up in China and helped us feel just a little bit closer to our future Chinese daughter.

However, there weren't many children's classes being offered on a Tuesday morning, but we did get to observe a pre-school age hip-hop dance class. All the little girls were dressed like pageant contestants in frilly tutus, sparkling dance shoes, and insanely large hair bows. The students were practicing a routine to Beyoncé's hit "Single Ladies," and popping their non-existent hips side to side. It was as ridiculous as it was adorable.

Watching the back-up dancers in training, made me miss my bi-weekly Zumba class. I fully credit Zumba (a workout phenomenon consisting of slightly naughty dance moves to hip-hop, reggaetón, and other popular Latin music) for keeping me sane throughout fertility treatments and the adoption process. My Swedish ancestors may have given me my height, blonde hair, and a passion for skiing but growing up in New Mexico gave me a Latin heart. I grew up listening to Mexican pop music and sneaking out of the house to go salsa dancing.

In addition to being insanely calorie-burning and incredibly stress-relieving, Zumba classes tend to have a wonderful mix of people and cultures. My Zumba classes always have numerous Asian dancers in bright colors, sometimes Indian women dancing in saris, randomly swirling hippies in long skirts, and a variety of stay-at-home-moms and suburban housewives in head-to-toe spandex. For a while, an older gentleman danced in the front row in various Navy T-shirts, blue jeans, and cowboy boots. There's always a mix of English, Spanish, Chinese, Hindi, and Tagalog (I had to inquire on this one).

I've always been athletic and used working out to relieve stress, but there's nothing like four years of infertility to turn you into a manic workout warrior. There were many times when I was so depressed, I sat in the bottom of my closet in the dark for hours; but then there were days when I was so filled with anxiety, I could have run a marathon on adrenaline alone.

I tried yoga and meditation but frequently failed to achieve any sort of stress relief or health benefit due to my jittery, nervous energy. Five minutes in, I was already looking at the clock. After ten minutes, my back hurt; after fifteen minutes, I began to feel like I needed to pee; and after twenty minutes, I was bored out of my damned mind and starting to nibble on my fingernails.

For me, during the worst days of torment, when my emotional roller coaster was about to derail, nothing beat really loud bomba music and shaking my ass. I was filled with way too much of the stress hormone cortisol to lie calmly in Savasana. If I wasn't attacking moguls with a maniacal intensity during the Colorado ski season, I was releasing pent-up frustration doing Zumba. I didn't have the patience to slowly foster a sense of well-being. I needed to work shit out!

On our last day in Shanghai, we took another, more enjoyable, walk around Renmin Park and Square.

The park was once the site of the Shanghai Race Club, established in 1862 by the British, and the height of Shanghai society in the early twentieth century. The area featured a horse racing track, a cricket pitch, and a swimming pool.

According to Daisy, "The club's flagpole was a great source of shame for the Chinese, as it was made from the mast of a Chinese warship captured by British and American troops. When the Communist Party took power in 1949, the new Chinese National Flag was hung from the pole to great celebration by the Chinese."

The Communist government quickly banned horse racing and gambling, as it was considered a symbol of Western decadence. Then, in 1952, the racetrack was converted into the People's Park (the northern half) and the People's Square (the southern half).

Without question, the most memorable aspect of the park was the Marriage Market, where parents advertised their children's availability for marriage and shopped for suitable sons- and daughters-in-law (or truth be told, grandparents auctioned off their grandkids). On the weekends, hundreds of marriage advertisements in plastic sheet protectors are strung up between trees and hung along walls with clothespins on lengths of twine like laundry—yet another version of Chinese National Flags.

Lucky for us, Daisy translated a couple of the advertisements:

Single Male. Bachelor's Degree. CPA. Born in 1973. 200,000 RMB a year. Looking for pretty girl who lives in the city.

Male. Born 1980. 1.8 m. Master's Degree. Shanghainese. Working in Fortune 500 Company. Looking for someone born between 1974 and 1982. Bachelor's degree or above.

There was even a large poster with a photograph of a Chinese nurse living in California who was searching for a Chinese husband willing to move to the United States.

Due to the one-child rule, many Chinese parents have only one child to care for them in their old age. Therefore, many believe the person their child marries bears great importance on how well they may hope to be cared for in their golden years. The phenomenon has become known as the 4-2-1 problem, in which only children must bear the responsibility of supporting both of their parents and, sometimes, all four of their grandparents in their old age, as they cannot rely on siblings to help them care for their aging family. Additionally, more than 40 million Chinese men may never find a wife, because they don't exist, leading grandma and grandpa to be a tad desperate and pushy.

While the success rate was notoriously low, the marriage bazaar swarmed with matchmaking hopefuls, rain or shine, every weekend. (And here I thought meeting my husband through Match.com was embarrassing. At least my grandparents didn't advertise my stats in a public park.)

I seriously considered asking Daisy if there was a Baby Market, where desperate, infertile couples could search for babies in need of a good home but feared it may not be an appropriate question in a country struggling with and being criticized for population-control measures.

Daisy told us that the senior citizens of Shanghai have their own dating scene at . . . IKEA! Apparently, ever since the Swedish department store began offering free coffee to holders of their family membership cards, anywhere from seventy to several hundred seniors flock to the Xuhui branch IKEA every weekend looking for love.

As we walked back toward our hotel, Daisy asked if we would like to "experience" a Shanghai subway station. She explained that she would never recommend that a foreigner travel by subway in China, but that visiting a subway station in Shanghai was an experience, and she wasn't wrong!

China's subway systems may be a cheap and convenient mode of travel but only if you have a death wish. We stopped for a short visit to the underground People's Square subway station, which was total bedlam! The ever-expanding Shanghai subway system has the longest route in the world at 334 miles (538 kilometers), while the Beijing metro system has the highest ridership. From what we observed, most aspects of life in major Chinese cities were cramped, but the subway cars looked more densely packed than a sardine can.

Daisy informed us that during college she had a part-time job, during peak subway rush hours, as a subway pusher. Her job was to force commuters' stray limbs and bulky carry-ons onto the train, so the doors could seal shut and the subway could be on its way (and for her efforts, she told us she regularly received a "blood nose").

While the subway was intimidating, it was even difficult just to cross a major intersection in Shanghai. When crossing from the People's Square to Nanjing Road, it was a tough call whether to walk through the chaotic underground subway station or line up on the street corner and cross the intersection blindly en masse.

In the time it took for a light to change at major intersections in Shanghai, easily fifty pedestrians (which felt more like a hundred from all the pushing and shoving) would gather to cross the street. Then, a massive swarm of people would push across the intersection, blindly moving with the force of the mob, like lemmings headed for an unknown cliff.

As a small-town girl, at least by China's standards, I had yet to fear for my life as a pedestrian. However, I quickly learned that when crossing major intersections in Beijing, Shanghai, and other large cities in China, one must tread very carefully or perish. Chinese drivers do not stop for pedestrians, follow standard traffic rules, or seem to care about designated lanes or crosswalks (and neither do those riding bikes and mopeds).

If you simply must cross a major intersection in China, be prepared to treat the endeavor as a contact sport. Expect to be jabbed in the ribs, unknown hands to touch your bum, and multiple shoes to crush your toes. Like a quarterback attempting to reach the end zone, your progress will be impeded by business executives, packs of teenagers, shoppers with personal wheeled carts, mothers pushing enormous baby strollers, and tiny but deadly senior citizens. Crossing major intersections in China's biggest cities was like navigating through football fans at a play-off game, spectators at Disneyworld when Cinderella makes her grand entrance, or the hallways of a typical American high school when the bell rings.

If you do not dispense with common courtesy and push your way through your fellow pedestrians, or at the very least stand your ground, you will go around in circles, get crushed, and likely never reach your destination. Best of luck!

For our last dinner in China, I'm embarrassed to admit that instead of having a traditional Chinese meal, utter exhaustion led us to a quick, easy, and cheap dinner at McDonald's.

As it turned out, the McDonald's located on the Nanjing Road pedestrian mall wasn't all that quick, easy, or cheap. There was a giant, walk-up counter with a row of eight cash registers and attendants; however, there was no ordering process, no cueing system, and absolutely no sense of procedure. One last time, we had to jump into the fray and get down and dirty Chinese-style using our only weapons: our superior height, my blonde hair, and our show-stoppingly unique Westerness.

We triumphantly ordered fast food in Shanghai (and it took only twenty minutes). The burgers had cucumbers, a spicy brown sauce, and much more flavorful beef; the french fries, however, were the same thin, limp, greasy strings we'd grown accustomed to in the States (and the yogurt parfait was as expected).

The evening ended on a high note with a fabulous Chinese acrobat performance. The show included a traditional lion dance, a magician, a contortionist, and multiple jugglers. The incredibly limber and agile performers juggled hats; tossed rolls on strings; jumped through hoops; contorted into tubes; rode motorbikes inside a giant metal ball; and otherwise jumped, flipped, twisted, and roller-skated in perfect unison.

In a truly grand finale, a tiny woman walked across the top of a row of six other women's heads, all while each of the women twirled flat plates on top of long thin sticks. Several of the gymnasts held four twirling sticks in each hand. Then, the woman on top flipped upside down, so she was head to head with another performer, all while twirling plates and not missing a beat. Plus, seven acrobats formed a variety of pyramids on top of another performer—as she steered a moving bicycle. It was insane!

As our time in Shanghai drew to a close, I had a new appreciation for home, my beloved colorful Colorado. I missed the temperate climate, cleaner air and relative wide-open spaces; a land where most everyone is an environmentalist, hardly anyone smokes, and people love to get outdoors; a place where our dogs are members of the family (not potential snacks).

But I had much to thank China for. I was returning home rejuvenated and full of positive qi. I learned a lot from a land where ancient traditions are still sacred, religion is not just a belief but a way of life, seniors are respected for their wisdom and guidance, good health involves balance within the whole body, and the people appreciate hard work and set high standards on education. Thanks to China, I had regained my thirst for learning, outgoing nature, and positive attitude.

As I wrote my final thoughts about Shanghai in the last remaining pages of my (second) journal, the night before leaving China, my pen ran out. It wasn't just any old pen. It was the pen, with green ink that smelled like apples that my favorite tour guide and friend Laura gave me at the start of our journey in Beijing.

"For the lady that is always asking questions and writing about China and who will one day become a mother to a Chinese baby," she had said on our last night together in Beijing.

I felt a heavy sadness as I realized how far we had come and that our journey through China was nearly at an end. I kept the useless pen in my journal, unwilling to part with it and its connection to my wonderful experiences in China.

It's not every day that a former small-town newspaper reporter turned elementary school teacher and a tech support specialist from Colorado have the opportunity to travel to China. With the goal to learn as much as possible about China, to become culturally aware and sensitive parents to an adopted Chinese child, we packed a lot into the once-in-a-lifetime trip. It was a whirlwind itinerary, from the historic cities of northern China to the beautiful countryside of southern China, we covered some serious ground, learned an incredible amount, and created lasting memories.

In the Shanghai airport, I allowed myself one last shopping spree, blowing our remaining Chinese yuan on last-minute souvenirs, then had to run to catch our plane. As I collapsed into my seat, loaded down with random trinkets and completely exhausted from travel, sick from the wet weather and worn down by the intense energy of China, I had a minor breakdown.

The full weight of returning home hit me like a ton of bricks. We had learned volumes about China and felt better prepared to become parents of a Chinese orphan, but we were returning home empty handed (besides the new suitcase full of Chinese folk art and fertility talismans). The harsh reality was that this was not *the* trip to China to receive our baby girl; it was simply a nice vacation. We were returning home to continue to wait, worry, and wonder when will we ever become parents?

For the millionth time, I wondered why I couldn't get or stay pregnant and asked the universe, "What's wrong with me?" "Am I too old, at thirty-five?" "Do I have some ultra-rare, impossible to detect, life-altering condition?"

I began to panic and question the adoption process, which had already taken too long. "Did our adoption agency lose our paperwork?" "Is the agency not legitimate?" "Did we miss the phone call or somehow get skipped on the waiting list?"

Most of all I questioned what I did to deserve this continuing hell. "Haven't I been a good person?" "Haven't I proved my love of children by dedicating my life to teaching?" "Am I cursed or being punished?"

Once more, I begged the universe to send me a sign, to answer the question, "Will I ever become a mother?"

While our trip to China was incredible, it was only a brief escape from our childless reality. Awaiting us back home were the stacks of books on adoption, the boxes of fertility drugs, the wastebasket full of negative pregnancy tests, the phone that continued to remain silent.

I quietly cried into the back of an inflatable travel pillow, swatting away my concerned husband, and ignoring the kind flight attendant trying to comfort me with a beverage. My tears seemed endless, like troubled waters I dare hoped had subsided but now flowed out of control.

I eventually passed out from both physical and emotional exhaustion and slept fourteen hours to Chicago.

Had our trip to China changed anything?

Anything at all?

16

AN UNEXPECTED PATH

Back home in Colorado, Chris and I enjoyed a wonderful reunion with our black and white, rescue, "fur baby" Otis.

The next day, the three of us celebrated with a long hike.

There's something about taking a long walk in the majestic mountains with your man and your dog.

For some time, Chris and I walked in silence, enjoying the blue sky and the breeze blowing through the aspens and the pines. After a while, we began to talk about the future. For the first time, we both admitted to our concerns about the adoption process and doubt that we would ever receive a Chinese child. We had been on the waiting list for two years and no tangible progress had been made.

The trail took us past an overlook, and we paused to peer into a vast gully and across to the other side where the terrain rose sharply, and boulders and pine trees mingled on the incline.

When we had left for China, we were broken. After two failed IVF attempts, I swore I would never go through the emotional and invasive experience again. Instead, I transferred all my hopes and dreams into adoption plans. The promise of a

Chinese baby had become my lifeline in a swirling sea of grief and loss.

Now, as we stood atop the summit, daring to admit that adoption may not be the answer and that we were no closer to having a family, we feared our trip to China had done nothing to improve our circumstances.

But China had improved me.

After my meltdown on the plane, I'd taken a hard look at myself.

While in China, I'd felt true joy, let go of emotional baggage, sought adventures, met interesting people, and smiled and laughed alongside my husband. I'd learned new things about the world, my marriage, and myself. I was more connected to my husband, and my marriage was stronger. My body felt heathier, my mind felt clearer, and my heart felt more at peace. I had become more emotionally grounded, spiritually aware, and open to new pathways.

I had rediscovered the long-forgotten woman who is outgoing, curious, and positive, and I never wanted to ignore or forget her again. More than anything I didn't want to go back to a life on hold, a life of longing and sadness.

Somehow, I knew that Chris and I were going to survive this battle and have a family.

I looked at Chris and said, "Let's give it one more try."

We found a new doctor and, two months after returning from China, I was diagnosed with an inherited gene mutation. While this mutation doesn't affect my daily life, it was potentially disrupting my ability to conceive and carry a pregnancy.

I have methylenetetrahydrofolate reductase or MTHFR. Of the many types of MTHFR mutations, I am homozygous C677T, placing me within the medium to high-risk factor.

The MTHFR gene creates the enzyme that breaks down the potentially toxic amino acid homocysteine. Those with this gene mutation often have elevated levels of homocysteine, which potentially increases the risk of neural tube defects and blood clots. Since babies receive oxygen via their mother's blood in-utero, any disruption to the blood flow due to a blood clot or poor circulation could lead to serious problems.

In addition, those with MTHFR gene mutations have a reduced ability to convert folate and B vitamins into a usable form. Basically, all those oh-so-important prenatal vitamins simply wash away with every trip to the ladies' room. And that's just the starting point for potential conception and pregnancy issues. There are also auto-immune conditions, mental disorders, and muscular conditions in those with severe MTHFR gene mutations and high homocysteine levels.

And adding insult to injury, the acronym for this disorder almost spells a swear word you might say when you first hear the diagnosis.

If you have suffered a miscarriage or are struggling to conceive, do yourself a favor and get a thrombophilia workup. Besides me, my half sisters, my best friend, her coworker, and a neighbor all have some form of the gene mutation. It's literally everywhere and likely to affect you or someone you love.

A century ago, it was considered normal for women to have at least one miscarriage. Today, as scientists and doctors work to better understand MTHFR, new medical technology and understanding is proving that often miscarriages need no longer be painfully accepted.

An early diagnosis of MTHFR might have saved me from years of severe depression, taking dangerous hormone drugs, throwing away nearly forty thousand dollars on potentially unnecessary fertility treatments, and a long and exasperating adoption process. Oddly enough, the man responsible for diagnosing my disorder and changing my life forever is named Dr. Bush!

The treatment for my MTHFR was a relatively simple protocol involving blood thinners. Sadly, Chris and I will never know if we could have gotten pregnant with the help of blood thinners alone, since at the age of thirty-six, we didn't have the luxury of time (nor the remaining patience or sanity) for experimentation. After more than four years of misery, it was a simple question of continuing trying to get pregnant naturally or start living our lives as parents. We finally had a clear diagnosis and a potential solution. So, with the aid of the blood thinning medication Lovenox and Dr. Bush, we tried a third round of IVF and got pregnant again.

I vividly remember one pivotal, terrifying day in the early stages of my pregnancy because it was both the worst and best day of my life.

We were in Santa Fe visiting my mother, who was recovering from breast cancer. Thankfully, doctors discovered the cancer early, and she avoided chemotherapy. But she was still suffering from the effects of surgery and radiation. Meanwhile, we were in the fragile, nerve-wracking early stage of another pregnancy attempt.

The day after we arrived, upon taking that typical early morning trip to the bathroom, I was horrified to see the toilet fill up with bright red blood. I screamed and sobbed and collapsed on the floor, and my poor mother came limping into the bathroom, clutching her arm against her breast.

The next four hours were a complete blur that started with a thirty-minute mad dash to the hospital to then sit and fret for nearly two hours in the ER waiting room. During the ultrasound, Chris and I heard a loud, clear heartbeat, which might have been comforting except for the fact that the heartbeat we were hearing might simply have been mine. We saw various peanut shaped blobs and desperately begged the ultrasound tech for information, but he pleaded the fifth and deferred to the doctor. So we waited another hour and a half for the doctor to visit and tell us the results of the ultrasound.

And so it was in the ER at St. Vincent Hospital in Santa Fe that we learned we had not miscarried again. We were still pregnant and that I was in fact carrying twins. This was the first time in our long journey that we learned that not one but two hearts were pumping. In every previous disappointment and loss we never even developed a heartbeat.

We hadn't miscarried. During the implantation process for two, a blood clot had developed and had simply bled out. Our two babies had strong heartbeats. But we still had a long road ahead of us.

When carrying twins, you literally count (and then celebrate) every hour that you continue "baking." Each week, day, hour, second is a huge milestone in a twin's pregnancy, as you struggle to make it to the full-term finish line or somewhere remotely close.

I spent the entire first half of my pregnancy terrified of having another miscarriage and the second half in constant fear of preterm labor. At each prenatal appointment, my heart raced, my hands shook, my legs were weak, and I whispered a silent plea, "Please be healthy, active . . . alive."

During the many long days and restless nights when I became crippled with fear and overcome with anxiety, I would look at my nightstand and see my collection of Chinese symbols of happy marriage, abundance, and luck and feel much needed comfort and courage.

As my belly quickly grew rounder, I worked on a scrapbook of photos and mementos from our trip to China, completed the One Hundred Good Wishes Quilt (with the inclusion of Chinese deadly animals), and began writing my memoir about the wonders of China and the many paths to motherhood. China was on my mind and in my heart every step of my pregnancy, helping to keep me calm, focused, and positive.

We were given a short reprieve from our constant pregnancy worries in the middle of the second trimester when I was at twenty-five weeks (call it the pregnancy sweet spot). This perfect mid-pregnancy timing happened to coincide with my birthday in October. We wanted to take a last-hurrah, birthday babymoon to Hawaii; but since I was classified as a high-risk pregnancy, the seven-hour flight was strictly prohibited. So, we took an hour-and-a-half flight to San Diego and enjoyed our last pre-kids vacation on the island of Coronado.

Throughout the years when I was unable to get and stay pregnant, one of my deepest desires was to lie on a beach in a bikini with a giant, pregnant belly. During our babymoon in San Diego, Chris took a picture of me, my tummy bursting out of a bikini, wearing a giant beach hat and smiling like the Cheshire cat.

As we drew nearer to my delivery date, the festivities began.

Less than a month before the twins were born, we held a traditional, Western, baby shower with a "two peas in a pod" theme. The party featured all the American standards, including the "guess what's in the diaper bag" game, pastel-colored decorations, gentle farm animal baby gifts, and carrot cake. I wore my favorite pink, floral, maternity maxi dress and was damn near bursting from the extra seventy pounds.

Three weeks later, the twins were born during a snowstorm in February. In the end, all I needed to carry a pregnancy to fruition was daily injections of blood thinners for a whopping ten-dollar copay a month to the local Walgreens. After a nearly forty-thousand-dollar investment, ingesting and injecting fertility drugs with horrible side effects, starting an international adoption, going to China and back, and suffering through five years of sheer hell, the key to motherhood was relatively simple, cheap, and painless. With the help of Lovenox, I carried our twins to thirty-seven weeks.

I have strong, albeit delirious, memories of heading toward an emergency C-section upon developing preeclampsia on a Tuesday evening and begging the OB to make sure my babies weren't born on a Wednesday (so they wouldn't be filled with woe like their mom). As it turns out, my twins are "full of grace."

I was finally, happily, overwhelmingly a mother of two: a girl and a boy.

Adoption was supposed to be our path to parenthood, and I think about and am grateful for our Chinese spirit baby every day because she gave us strength, comfort, and faith. But in the end, a medical diagnosis led to us finally becoming parents. While it may have been technical and untraditional, I got to grow life (or lives) inside of me, and for that I'm forever grateful to modern science.

Since I'd waited five long, hard years to celebrate the birth of a child and ended up with twins, I decided to have two baby showers instead of one.

To honor the spirit of our Chinese baby who gave us the hope of a child, and to celebrate our twins' first one hundred days, we hosted a customary Chinese Red Egg and Ginger Party.

In China, a baby's first month is celebrated with hard-boiled eggs dyed red and pickled gingerroot. Eggs are considered lucky since they represent fertility, birth, and life, while red is the color of happiness and good luck. Ginger symbolizes a family's deep roots and the perpetuation of family lineage.

According to the Chinese, a new mother is cool, since her qi is considered full of yin after childbirth. Therefore, a new mother's internal balance of yin and yang needs to be restored. The key ingredient to warming a mother's body and increasing her strength is ginger.

At one month old, a Chinese child celebrates many firsts, including the first bath, the first fancy outfit, and the first haircut. Customarily, parents would shave the baby's head, except for the top of the crown, to remove the hair grown in the womb and encourage new growth. The baby hair was then tied with a red ribbon or placed in a red pouch and kept as a keepsake. However, I wasn't about to cut my daughter's nearly non-existent peach fuzz, blonde hair. (For the first three years, everyone thought I had twin boys).

Traditionally, at one month, a Chinese baby's birth is officially announced, the child is presented to the ancestors, and he or she is given a name. We chose complimentary names from Norse mythology months in advance and sent out hundreds of birth announcements with a pear motif and the line "A Perfect Pair" within a week of the twins' birth. We had waited long enough and our time to celebrate and announce our parenthood to the world was overdue!

These days Chris and I live in a monotonous world of laundry, running errands, and cleaning up after kids and their variety of pets. Typical days now involve carting the twins to the children's museum, swim lessons, and Costco in a muddy, Cheerios-and-dog-fur covered (but bumper sticker-free) Honda Pilot.

We're lucky if we get two to three date nights a year, are way too exhausted for a robust sex life, and dream of the day when our kids are old enough to attend sleep-away camp, so we can finally take a relaxing vacation (or just watch Netflix and sleep). Not that I'm complaining, although there are days when I hide in my closet in the dark again, immobilize the kids in car seats and drive around aimlessly belting my heart out to Adele, and steal all their animal crackers and dip them in Nutella.

But then there are those sweet and tender moments when the twins reach out to hold my hands as I walk them to school, ask to climb into bed with me in the mornings, and ask for "bunny, elephant, squish and mega" kisses at night. Plus, who wouldn't love a stick figure portrait of "Mume" with yellow hair that reaches the ground, giant circle knees, and enormous red nails— not to mention spontaneous dance parties, macaroni necklaces, woven potholders and pinecone sculptures, and family-themed Halloween costumes?

Even after the toughest days of parenting (the nonstop bickering in the car, full meltdowns in public places, and "you're mean because you make me eat vegetables, won't buy me a cellphone, don't let me play video games all day" rants), I always tuck my kids into bed, read them books, sing songs, including

"Summertime," give them hugs and kisses, and tell them how much I love them. All this because I will never forget how much it hurts to have a father who never hugged or said I love you, a stepfather who made me feel like an unwanted burden, and a stepmother who betrayed my trust and ruined my relationship with my family.

But most of all, I'll never forget how hard we fought, how much we suffered, and how long we wished to become parents. And I will never take motherhood for granted.

꧁

According to an ancient Chinese legend, a god ties an invisible red cord around the ankles of those that are destined to meet. The deity responsible for the Red Thread of Fate is the old lunar matchmaker god in charge of marriages, Yuè Lǎo. However, there are many in the adoption world that believe a red thread also attaches future parents to their destined child. Somewhere along the line, the magical red cord attaching us to a Chinese orphan—which supposedly never breaks—managed to sever. Our adoption of a baby girl from China will likely never come to pass.

Officially, we are *still* on the waiting list—ten years and counting—with no end in sight. Shortly after returning from China, the Chinese government put an end to the one-child rule, grinding the international adoption program to a halt. The Chinese population was becoming male dominated and elderly, and the workforce was beginning to shrink. The one-child policy began to phase out in 2015, and on January 1, 2016, a new law allowing for two children for all Chinese people, regardless of minority group, came into effect.

In addition, China had long been criticized for its strict adoptive parent requirements, which go above and beyond the typical income standards to include an age and weight limit. Sadly, singles, older couples, the entire LGBTQ community, people with a high body mass index, and those who can't pay the price need not apply.

Both my husband and I entered our forties after our fifth year on the waiting list. So essentially, we are no longer qualified for an adoption program that has basically ceased to exist. Americans would say it's a lost cause, while the Chinese might say *yuan mù qiú yú*, which means "climbing a tree to catch a fish."

We will never take a trip to the fabled Baby Island or Shamian Island, the location of the American Consulate in Guangzhou, where most American couples adopting Chinese babies got their child's visa. There will never be a stay at the White Swan Hotel in Guangzhou, known as the White Stork Hotel, where new parents were given a gift basket of baby supplies. (There was a Mattel sponsored play area, and packs of babies tottered about the pink marble lobby.) There will be no legendary red couch photo (a tradition where each adoption group gathered with their new babies on a red couch in the hotel lobby for an official photograph).

The initial purpose of our trip to China—to become culturally educated and sensitive adoptive parents to a future Chinese orphan—was for naught; however, the trip itself was not in vain.

My trip to China saved me from depression, boosted my faith, rekindled my hope, and made me feel reborn. As frustrating, painful, and expensive as my journey to motherhood proved to be, if I hadn't gone through fertility treatments and the adoption process, I likely never would have taken a life-changing trip to China, the effects of which still benefit and enrich me today.

So if you're struggling to survive one of life's many challenges and depression is kicking in, I highly recommend traveling. It will likely save your sanity, improve a relationship, and help you on your journey. Try out a new persona, let go of old burdens, meet some new people, seek out adventures, learn new things about the world, and reconnect with yourself.

For those of you dealing with infertility, why not make all those obnoxiously happy families sending you regular birth announcements and holiday cards jealous by sending them photos of crystal blue waters and white sandy beaches? And while you're relaxing in the sun, drink as many piña coladas as you damned well please. (Then jump in the sack out of spontaneous, wanton lust. It may or may not get you pregnant, but who cares when you're actually having some fun.)

Once children enter the picture, the concept of a vacation, where you return rested, relaxed, and refreshed with a tan, ceases to exist. You trade exotic international and therapeutic spa vacations for trips to grandma's house and Legoland (all while lugging diapers, car seats, and a stroller).

For us, travel was the key to surviving years of infertility. Breaking free from our obsession with pregnancy and constant reminders of our childlessness to completely immerse ourselves in another world, gave us a momentary reprieve from crushing depression, anxiety, and pain. For a brief moment, we could change our course, alter our reality, and live a completely new, exciting, and happy life.

In life's crazy, unpredictable, maddening way, I went from being frustrated and confused by not getting pregnant naturally; depressed and anxious while undergoing fertility treatments; distraught and sick from failures and losses; hopeful and enthusiastic for adoption of a Chinese orphan; shocked and scared by a medical diagnosis; excited but terrified by a twin's pregnancy; and finally happy and thankful to be a mother of two. Looking back at my five-year journey to motherhood and its numerous paths, it feels like I lived entirely different lives.

We desperately try to influence the direction of our lives but often find we have little control when fate steps in with other plans and sets us on an entirely different course. While a new path may not be what we planned or hoped for, it's sure to be a learning experience with new adventures, which hopefully don't involve eating a dog.

China will always be an important part of my family's life. I continue to read books about Chinese history, culture, and tradition; follow the art of feng shui; and tutor Asian immigrants. Our generic suburban home is now filled to bursting with Chinese folk art, antiques, and travel mementos. Our family celebrates several Chinese holidays and attends local Chinese festivals. Plus, we eat store-bought dumplings on a regular basis.

As incredible as it sounds, my twins were born in the middle of February, during Chinese New Year and the Year of the Tiger; so I literally am a tiger mom. As Gold Tigers, my children are both independent and boldly express themselves. By complete chance, the kids are learning Mandarin at our neighborhood grade school and bring home plastic straw abacuses, Chinese calligraphy, and brush stroke panda paintings.

If I am ever fortunate enough to return to China, hopefully with my family beside me, I would love to sit on a park bench in Tiantan or Beihai Park in Beijing, drink green tea, and watch the locals play chess, practice calligraphy, and fly kites. Maybe I'd even join them. In Hangzhou, I would enjoy a casual stroll around West Lake, and a day of contemplation at the Temple of the Soul's Retreat. I would relish a peaceful afternoon of writing and sketching in my journal under a willow tree on Love Island in Guilin with a view of Elephant Trunk Hill. Most of all, I would cherish another trip down the Li River to Yangshuo, this time on a tiny bamboo raft, to continue my search for dragons.

I will forever keep the spirit of my Chinese baby in my upper heart. For this baby that was never destined to be mine, gave me comfort, renewed my faith, and healed my heart. It's not an exaggeration to say that my spirit baby and the country of China saved me, because they did. The prospect of a Chinese baby girl and our amazing trip to China pulled me back from the edge of despair, helped me to become more vital and positive, and guided me along my journey to motherhood.

My once broken and empty heart is now filled with a profound and deep love for the incredible country of China, my amazing family, and my unforgettable spirit baby. This book of my wonderful memories of China, is my small gift to you, spirit baby, with gratitude and love.

Thank you. Xièxiè. 谢谢

EPILOGUE

As full and complete as our life has become, there is always room for unexpected insights and gifts.

Recently, I took the twins to an air show at the local municipal airport. As we wandered through the rows of planes, I shared a sentimental memory of my father, who passed away when they were just ten months old.

I told them how my father loved to fly. He would take me to air shows every summer, drone on and on about the history and types of planes, and quiz me on the aeronautical alphabet. My father became a different person while piloting a plane, excited and happy like a kid at Christmas. These special moments are my fondest recollection of him.

As I pointed out an old Cessna and told my children about the serial number on grandpa's plane (N4868Y), I suddenly burst into tears. Revisiting this happy childhood memory and fondly remembering my father led me to realize that my childhood loneliness and isolation are finally over.

I am a mother, I have a family, and I belong.

ABOUT THE AUTHOR

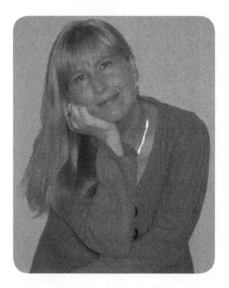

Nina Neilson Little is a mountain-town newspaper reporter, turned magazine editor, turned early childhood literacy teacher, turned author of books for adults and children. Having grown up in eccentric Santa Fe, New Mexico, she loves the arts and anything Latin: food, music and especially dancing. No longer the world traveler, she enjoys ski trips and the occasional vacation to the beach with her family. She lives in a former mining town turned suburb in the foothills of Colorado with her husband, boy/girl twins, two large mutts and a pompous bearded dragon.

To follow the author and view photos of China, please visit http://www.ninalittlebooks.com.